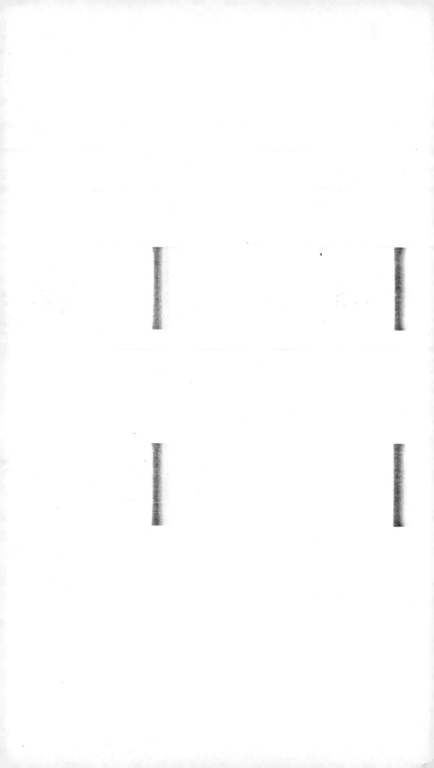

# How Much
# Does Your Soul
# Weigh?

Also by Dorie McCubbrey, M.S.Ed., Ph.D.

*Dr. Dorie's "Don't Diet" Book*

# How Much Does Your Soul Weigh?

DIET-FREE SOLUTIONS
TO YOUR FOOD, WEIGHT,
AND BODY WORRIES

Dorie McCubbrey, M.S.Ed., Ph.D.

HarperResource
*An Imprint of* HarperCollins*Publishers*

This book is not intended to substitute for the advice of a medical professional. If your weight and other problems are causing you to be physically ill or are preventing you from functioning normally on a daily basis, you should seek the advice of the appropriate medical professional. The names of certain individuals have been changed to protect their privacy.

HarperCollins books may be purchased for educational, business, or sales promotional use. For information please write: Special Markets Department, HarperCollins Publishers Inc., 10 East 53rd Street, New York, NY 10022.

FIRST EDITION

*Designed by Nancy Singer Olaguera*

Library of Congress Cataloging-in-Publication Data

McCubbrey, Dorie.
    How much does your soul weigh : diet-free solutions to your food, weight, and body worries / Dorie McCubbrey.—1st ed.
        p. cm.
    Includes bibliographical references.
    ISBN 0-06-621375-4
        1. Weight loss—Psychological aspects. 2. Eating disorders—
    Psychological aspects.  I. Title.

RM222.2 .M4338 2002
613.7'01'9—dc21

                                                                2002068728

03 04 05 06 07 ❖/QW 10 9 8 7 6 5 4 3 2

For Shadow
*See the Light*

# contents

# ～ acknowledgments

I would like to express my gratitude to the many souls who helped this book "come to life." Joann Davis, you sparked the initial concept, working with me to express my soul's wisdom in written form. You are an extraordinary literary agent, and it has been such a blessing to work with you! Jennifer Brehl, your editorial brilliance has enhanced the flow of the words of my soul, and you truly have guided this book to "be born." I have thoroughly enjoyed our connection on this project!

There are hundreds of clients whom I have had the privilege to help over the years. I have learned so much from all of you, and now others can, too. Your voices can be heard throughout this book, giving encouragement for all on their journey of freedom. I am especially thankful to the Reverend Jack Groverland and everyone at Unity of Boulder, where I held my first "How Much Does Your Soul Weigh?" workshops. Jack, your soulful wisdom is a light on the path for us all.

I would also like to acknowledge my colleagues who carefully reviewed my manuscript, offering much soulful feedback: Dr.

Linda Harper, Dr. Anita Johnston, the Reverend Cindy LeVeque, Carolyn Pickler, Heather Guthrie, Kasey McCullough, Amy Skolon, Mary Casey, Paige Glass, and John Ensign. I express my deepest gratitude to you all. Sandra Ford Walston, you have given me such encouragement to move forward—courageously—as an author and speaker! I also thank you and Marianne Naples for connecting me with my agent—the synchronicity is awesome. Mark Camacho, your video production and marketing expertise helped me to clarify and focus my message. I'm especially grateful for the "mirror." I would also like to thank my many other colleagues in the National Speakers Association, and especially my local chapter in Colorado. You have all helped me to strengthen the voice of my soul.

Mom and Dad, I couldn't have done it without you! Thank you for the gift of life, and for all your support over the years. My brother Doug, our journeys have so many parallels—let's keep moving forward on the path. My brother David, you have helped me to realize what an asset the "engineer in me" can be. Jeff Rogers, thank you for believing in me always. Pico and Miler, I cherish your unconditional love and companionship. Many thanks to my friends for your insights, enthusiasm, and kindness, especially Chanin Walsh, Patricia Rose Upczak, Tom Oginsky, Julie Chiravelli, Kamala Tran, Janice Hoffman, Denise Zainia, Gary Cage, and all the folks at the Mountain Sun. I would also like to express my gratitude for the beautiful mountains and wilderness, where I always feel such connection and inspiration, keeping my soul light and free. Thank You, God!

# How Much
# Does Your Soul
# Weigh?

# your journey

## begins within

*How much does your soul weigh?*

When I ask that question, you may be wondering, "Well, what's my soul supposed to weigh? What *is* my soul, anyway? And what does my *soul's* weight have to do with solving my *body's* weight problem?" These are valid responses. After all, you've probably read countless books about eating and weight issues, and none have mentioned your soul. *That's because this book is vastly different from traditional approaches to weight control.* Most focus on "getting rid of" excess weight or eating disorders. However, these are just symptoms. *To become free of eating and weight problems requires addressing their cause.* You will not find the solution in any diet, meal plan, lifestyle change, or behavior modification program. Those regimens are all imposed from the outside. *The answers you seek are within.* This book will guide you from your body to your mind, and then from your mind to your soul—you

1

will discover how to solve your food, weight, and body worries from the inside out. It's no coincidence that you have started to read this book. A friend may have recommended it. You may have picked it off the shelf at a bookstore. It may have just "shown up." Whatever the means, the reason is that you are ready. Your soul is ready to help you. Are you aware of its presence?

*How much does your soul weigh?*

My soul is light and free. But it wasn't always this way. For many years, I had no awareness of my soul. All that mattered was my body. I was just like the 50 percent of women and 20 percent of men who worry about their weight some or all of the time. I joined the 100 million Americans who are trying to lose weight on any given day. Like 10 million Americans, my weight worries led to obsession and ultimately anorexia and bulimia. At the other extreme, I was also like 55 percent of the American population now considered to be overweight or obese. My attitude vacillated between total obsession with weight loss and complete apathy manifested by an "I don't care any more" attitude. My body suffered from starvation and binge eating, compulsive exercise and a sedentary lifestyle, repeated cycles of weight loss and weight gain. I was so worried about how much my body weighed. *But how much did my soul weigh?* I finally realized that for more than fifteen years I had been completely ignoring my soul, and that it felt extremely weighed down, buried under my ongoing emphasis on weight control. *Weight control was controlling me.* This was the real "weight" I needed to lose—my weight consciousness. This book is about a different kind of weight loss—about losing the "weight" that's burdening your soul, losing the "weighty attitudes" of the diet mentality.

*How much does your soul weigh?*

Does your soul feel weighed down by all your focus on weight control? Do you even know that you have a soul? Are you living your dreams and fulfilling your purpose in life? Or are you living a diet nightmare? Do you see yourself as a congruent extension of your core essence? Or has weight control been controlling you so much that you have forgotten who you really are and what is really important? Your symptoms are your teachers. Binge eating, purging, restrictive dieting, fasting, starving. Compulsive exercise, sedentary lifestyle. Overweight, underweight. These symptoms all have a message for you. Can you hear it? Or are you too busy trying to "get rid of" your symptoms to discover what they have to tell you? Maybe there is an issue you need to resolve in a current relationship. Or an issue from a past relationship. What about your relationship with your career or your finances? When you dig deep enough, you'll discover that it's all about your relationship with your soul. Your symptoms are a reflection of the "hunger from your soul"—an insatiable hunger, which binge eating cannot satisfy nor starvation deny. *To satisfy your soul's hunger, you need to give it your attention.* Wake up from your diet nightmare with the awareness of your soul. Listen to its voice. Honor its wisdom. Be its life.

*How much does your soul weigh?*

Your soul can be light and free. You can be who you really are, living in happiness, health, balance, peace, and confidence. You can achieve this success using *Intuitive Self-Care*—a process that I discovered and used to end my own fifteen-year struggle with eating disorders and weight problems. Now, as a licensed professional counselor, an author and professional speaker, I continue to use this process to maintain my freedom and to guide thousands on their journey of freedom. This book includes three sections, which address *why* the games dieters play don't work, *what* the process of Intuitive Self-Care is all about, and *how* you can apply this process to your life by nourishing your soul. You will learn the details of my own elusive quest for weight control, and how I discovered the solution within myself. You will discover the secrets of people who have never had weight problems, and the insights you need to reclaim your intuition, your spiritual birthright. You will experience the therapeutic benefits of my 30-day plan of "recipes" to feed your soul. Throughout the text, my clients (whose names have been changed to maintain confidentiality) will share their perspectives about their own journeys of freedom. In addition, I have included detailed case studies of the four archetypal weight problems, so that you can follow along the journey of freedom with the archetype that you most resemble. Within each chapter, you will have the opportunity to answer introspective questions, much like those I ask my clients during their sessions with me. This book is designed to be interactive, guiding you to find your own answers from within yourself. I encourage you to write your responses in a journal, instead of just thinking about them in your head. You can also use your journal to note your insights and to document your progress as you follow this program. Let your journal be a record of your journey of freedom.

*How much does your soul weigh?*

Are you ready to make the shift from focusing on how much your body weighs to how much your soul weighs? Are you ready to begin a new journey of freedom, with experiences more spectacular than you can imagine? Freedom is not about losing weight or getting rid of an eating disorder. These external symptoms may dissipate as a result of your freedom, but freedom begins *within*. Freedom is about *gaining* something—an awareness of your soul.

As you journey within yourself to this awareness, you will enjoy freedom. As I write this introduction, I am sitting on the summit of Green Mountain, at 8100 feet above sea level. I can see for miles, with a clarity that is not possible when I am "in the world" at lower elevations. The city of Boulder, Colorado is behind me. The wilderness of the Rocky Mountains is before me. This is a little bit what your journey of freedom will be like, and my clients and I will be your guide. You will be "rising above the world" to gain a new perspective, leaving the diet mentality behind you and moving forward to embrace your intuition, the voice of your soul. In a newsletter that I read recently, the actor Alan Alda said, "You have to leave the city of your comfort and go into the wilderness of your intuition. What you will discover will be wonderful. What you will discover will be yourself."

*How much does your soul weigh?*

Let your soul be light and free. But what if you've been struggling with weight issues for ten, fifteen, twenty or more years— you may wonder, can you truly be free? What if it feels as if your soul is hidden in total darkness—can you really find that light? I believe that freedom is possible for everyone. In fact, I view everyone as already free. *We just need to remember who we really are.* I received a phone call one morning at the crack of dawn from a woman who had been struggling for twenty-one years with weight problems and eating disorders. Given the early hour of her call, she seemed surprised that I answered the phone—her call for help. She spoke in the voice of the diet nightmare, the voice I knew so well, the only voice I used to be able to hear. And I responded to her in the voice of the soul, a voice that I was painfully aware she could not hear within herself. I asked her name, and she replied, "I don't want to give you my real name, but people call me Shadow." An appropriate name, given that she spoke in a voice of such darkness and despair. But by the end of our conversation I sensed that she was beginning to see a ray of light amidst the darkness. After I hung up the phone, I realized that this book is for Shadow. I found myself writing this book as if I were speaking to the Shadow part of myself, the part that had lived the diet nightmare and the part that still feels that pain. I wrote what I know I needed to hear in order to become free, and what I still need to hear in order to stay free. May the words upon these pages be the hope for Shadows everywhere. May these words, the voice of my soul and others' souls, help you hear the voice of your own soul. May you see beyond the darkness. *Shadow, see the Light . . .*

*Soulfully,*
*Dr. Dorie*
*Boulder, Colorado*

# Section I

~~

# Diet Dilemmas

# living the

## diet nightmare

I remember very clearly when my weight problem began. I was ten years old, and I was reading a story about a little girl who was always teased because she was fat. "How awful that would be," I thought. The girl described how her thighs rubbed together on hot summer days. Panic set in as I realized my thighs rubbed together too. "Maybe *I'm* fat," I thought. Although I was an average-sized child, this triggered my first diet. For the next fifteen years, my life revolved around weight control, and I experienced a variety of weight problems and eating disorders.

## THE QUEST TO FIT IN

Terrified of being teased because I was fat like that girl in the story, I decided I needed to be thin to be accepted by others. I compared my best friend's thighs to mine. Hers didn't rub together. Comparing her overall shape and size to mine, I noticed that I was much bigger all over. For the first time in my life I really started to *feel* fat. I went home and complained to my parents about being fat. My father, meaning well, said, "You're not fat, but you do have a nice little shelf," as he patted me on the butt. That confirmed it. I definitely was *fat!* My butt looked like a *shelf!* In my mind I saw a big fat shelf sticking out from the rear of my body. I didn't want to *stick out* and be teased— I wanted to *fit in* and be accepted. Losing weight seemed like the only solution.

*What kinds of messages did you get about your body as a child, and throughout your life? When did you first start to believe that you had to lose weight to fit in?*

## THE QUEST FOR ATTENTION

Although my parents were not dieters, they believed that dieting was acceptable and, in fact, necessary if someone was overweight. My father, a physician, often prescribed diets in his medical practice, and praised his patients who lost weight. My aunt and my sister-in-law were dieting, and I noticed that as they lost weight they received attention and compliments. My parents didn't see any harm in letting me watch what I ate, using my aunt and sister-in-law as role models. I started reading articles about diets and weight loss. I made changes in what and how much I was eating so I could lose weight. I started to exercise more. At first, these changes seemed healthy to my family, and I was getting positive attention for them. My parents noticed. My two older brothers noticed. My friends noticed. So, I figured, if a little was good, more would be better.

*Who in your life gave attention to others for their weight loss efforts? How did these people influence your dieting behaviors?*

## THE QUEST TO BE LIKED

While getting a positive reaction from my family and friends felt good, I *really* wanted that same positive reaction from the boys at school. I was attending a new middle school in my hometown of Plymouth, Michigan, and I wanted to be popular. The prettiest and thinnest girls seemed to be the best-liked, so I figured I had to be thin if I were ever to have a boyfriend. My mom, a home-maker, would always say, "It's what's inside that counts, but it sure helps to look good, too." She praised my internal qualities, but she also emphasized looks. She would often warn me, "People who are overweight have it so much harder." I thought again about the girl in that story, and how she was teased all the time. I wanted the boys to *like* me, not tease me. Thinness seemed the way to assure I'd be liked.

*Have you ever felt that being attractive on the inside wasn't enough? Have you ever been teased for your looks or your weight? How did you handle this?*

## THE QUEST TO COPE WITH A TRAUMA

In the sixth grade, I had to do a class presentation about the judicial system. I researched the project and came up with a fun and creative way to present the material. I dressed up the way I thought a lawyer would dress, and made my presentation to the class, pretending to be an attorney. Midway through, I was interrupted by my teacher, who mistook my dramatic style. "You obviously didn't take this seriously," she said. I was mortified. She continued with her criticism as the class laughed at me. I had been constructively criticized before by teachers, parents, and peers, but never destructively criticized like this. It was especially traumatic for me because I was at a critical developmental stage, moving from childhood into adolescence. I was just beginning to form a sense of my own identity, and my teacher's judgment was a crushing blow to my emerging self-image. Thinking I was flawed at my core, I could feel myself trying to shrink from sight. From that day forward, I was terrified to make a mistake. I no longer trusted my own inner guidance; instead, I looked outside myself for the approval of others. Weight control began to serve a powerful role—it symbolically let me "shrink" as a means of coping with my classroom humiliation.

*Some traumas seem minor on the surface but have a major impact, as in my example. Can you identify some of these "minor" traumas in your own life? What about major traumas, such as the death of a family member, abandonment by a significant person, or physical, emotional, or sexual abuse? How did your weight loss behaviors change in relation to any of these traumas?*

## THE QUEST TO COMPETE

The majority of my sixth-grade classmates were on diets, competing with each other to be the thinnest. It seemed as if it was the norm to try to lose weight. It was sort of a contest to see who could eat the least, who could fast the longest, who could exercise the hardest, and who could be the thinnest. So I began an all-out effort to be the thinnest. I cut my food intake to fewer than 600 calories per day. I exercised for hours, riding my bike, running up and down the stairs, or doing leg lifts. I cut out desserts and eliminated caloric beverages. I stopped eating after 6:00 P.M. I came up with a creative reason why I should be allowed to eat dinner alone in my room, and then I hid my food instead of eating it. If forced to eat at the dinner table with my family, I would secretly slip food from my mouth into my napkin, then throw it away. I asked for money to buy lunches at school, but never actually ate. Whenever I felt hungry, I denied the hunger and drank a diet cola instead. I took diet pills to numb my appetite even further. I cooked elaborate meals for my family, but ate only a few bites myself. I dropped weight dangerously fast. *Although I was thin, I still thought I was fat. I had become anorexic.* Anorexia Nervosa is an eating disorder characterized by low body weight, distorted body image, extremely restrictive eating, and compulsive exercise patterns.

*Has weight loss ever been a competition for you? Who did you compete with? Have you ever participated in a corporate weight loss program or a team weight loss? How did this competition affect you?*

## THE QUEST TO BE IN CONTROL

My parents, in a panic, did everything they could think of to get me to eat and gain weight. They didn't understand that my eating disorder was not about eating, and my weight problem was not about weight. They took me to doctors, and threatened to put me into a hospital where I would be fed through a tube if I didn't eat. All of this terrified me, making me feel even more out of control, resulting in a renewed resolution to control my weight. Weight became the one thing I could control when other aspects of my life felt out of control. I continued playing games with my food to convince my parents I was eating, when in fact I was still hiding food and skipping meals. There was no way I was going to let anyone force me to eat, because I was convinced I was still so *fat!*

*What has seemed out of control in your life? How have your weight loss behaviors given you a sense of being in control?*

## THE QUEST FOR WEIGHT MAINTENANCE

I continued with my rigid control, but then one day toward the end of my sixth-grade school year I remember feeling physically exhausted. I knew I was losing weight, but I wondered what could cause such an extreme lack of energy—unless I had lost more weight than I realized? I looked in the mirror at my naked body and was surprised to see it in its emaciated reality. I was not fat; I could see every rib clearly. *They were right! I was anorexic after all!* This experience of seeing my starving body scared me into eating. Physiologically and psychologically I had been starving, and now it seemed as if I couldn't get enough to eat. My body needed nutrients and my mind needed to overcome its deprivation. But I went from one extreme to the other, from anorexia to binge eating. I gorged on all the foods I had been denying myself. It was not uncommon for me to eat the majority of a coffee cake or a quart of ice cream at one sitting. I didn't worry about how much I was eating, because I was willing to gain *some* weight. But when I reached the weight at which I wanted to stay, *I was unable to stop gaining.* I rapidly regained all the weight I had lost, and then some. I became extremely depressed as I now felt fat all over again. I began the weight loss games again, in a quest to get back down to my ideal weight. But I was unable to reclaim the rigid control I had had as an anorexic. No matter what I tried, I couldn't even get close to that ideal weight. The reductions in my food intake and increases in my exercise were not enough—I just kept gaining.

*Have you ever experienced a period of deprivation followed by a period of binge eating? Have you ever reached your "goal weight," then been unable to maintain it? How did you handle this situation?*

## THE QUEST FOR HEALTH

Because my parents suspected that problems at school had triggered my anorexia, they decided that I should switch schools for the seventh grade. At my new school—a small private school in Ann Arbor, Michigan—very few of the girls were overly concerned about their weight. This lifted some of the pressure I had felt, but I continued to compare myself to the other girls, and weight control remained important to me. My focus shifted from losing weight to "just eating healthy and exercising," which, as I learned in my health class, was where the emphasis truly belonged. I followed "healthy diets" from magazines, tried special "healthy recipes" and food combinations, and tried to "eat healthy" by watching my fat intake. I joined sports teams to burn calories with "healthy exercise," and played various other weight loss games that I believed were "healthy." *But was I really being healthy, or was I being overly restrictive?* I was using "health" as a mask to cover unhealthy weight loss attempts.

*Have you tried to lose weight for health reasons? Have your weight loss attempts ever compromised your health? Have your "healthy" weight loss attempts actually been unhealthy?*

## THE QUEST TO BE THE BEST

In high school, a friend of mine was the star of the field hockey team, always scoring goals and making headlines in the local paper. One of my classmates was an excellent violinist and was the "concertmistress," the prestigious title given to the woman holding the first chair of the violin section. Another classmate always got straight A's, and ended up being the valedictorian. Meanwhile, I wasn't the best at *anything*. I was a field hockey player, but never in the limelight. I was a violinist, but never first chair. I did well in school, but never made straight A's. I felt that I was mediocre at everything. I yearned to be the best at *something*. I even felt like a failure at weight loss, but I figured that this was still my best shot to be the best at something. So I kept playing more weight loss games, searching for the one that would lead to my success.

*Have you ever been the best at something? What did you wish you could have been better at, or even the best? Has weight control given you the opportunity to be the best at something?*

## THE QUEST FOR SECURITY

As I encountered more teenage pressures, I turned to food as a means to cope. Food offered comfort, security, escape, and a temporary means to soften the sting of problems I was struggling with. Food had a strong, almost drug-like appeal. The more I ate, the better I felt—temporarily. But then I had to deal with the consequences of my eating—the fullness and the weight gain. If I had been addicted to drugs, my treatment would have been to abstain from them. But what about food? I couldn't just abstain from food. *I had to eat. But how could I eat without overeating?* I was becoming afraid of food, because it seemed as if once I started to eat I couldn't stop. I was still concerned about controlling my weight, but wasn't able to. I exercised to burn off the calories I had eaten, but continued to gain weight. All my years of dieting had slowed my metabolism, making it easier to put on the pounds. The more I gained, the more depressed I felt, and the more I turned to food to cope. My mom ended up going with me to a weight loss program at a local hospital. It addressed the emotional aspects of weight issues, and emphasized using portion control and other behavior modifications to control eating. However, this was just a "diet in disguise," serving as yet another weight loss game.

*What situations in your life have left you craving comfort or security? How have your patterns with eating, exercise or weight control satisfied this desire? Have you ever felt afraid of food, or that you might be "addicted" to it?*

## THE QUEST TO ESCAPE

Behind all of the weight loss efforts were underlying issues I wasn't even aware of. As long as I focused on weight control, I didn't have to face these issues. I was wearing many masks, trying to be what I thought others expected me to be. The perfect daughter. The perfect friend. The perfect student. All of these masks were layered on top of my core essence, so ultimately I didn't even know who I really was. In addition, all of the weight loss games I played were masks, each one designed to get my body to look a certain way. Weight control was an attempt to be who I thought I should be—but it was also an attempt to cope with the pain of not being who I really was. Eating, exercise, and weight control became the means by which I tried to escape from the pain of this inner turmoil, and to avoid other difficult issues.

*Can you identify specific conflicts in your life, or issues that you may be trying to avoid? How does weight control help you escape them?*

## THE QUEST FOR IMPROVED ATHLETIC PERFORMANCE

I attended The University of Michigan, where I played on the varsity field hockey team. This was rewarding, but it also fed into my desire to be thin. We were weighed on a regular basis, and if we gained weight we were reprimanded. One year, at the beginning of a new season after gaining weight over the summer, I was not placed in the starting lineup. The majority of my teammates had eating disorders, a fact that was virtually ignored by the athletic staff. In fact, one anorexic teammate was praised for her "extra efforts," showing up early to run laps and staying afterward to run even more. Even though she lacked strength, likely due to her inadequate nutrition, she had incredible endurance and we were all encouraged to "be like her."

*Sports like running, gymnastics, dancing, and wrestling place a high emphasis on weight. What sports have you played, and what were the messages you received about weight? How do you think weight is related to peak performance?*

## THE QUEST FOR THE IDEAL STANDARD

I visualized an ideal body that I hoped to achieve, based on the images that I saw in women's fashion and fitness magazines. I yearned to have a toned, cellulite-free, beautiful body like the models who graced the pages of all those magazines. I made a collage of pictures cut from magazines, showing ideal bodies and headlines like "Building A Beautiful Body" and "Instant Body Slimming" to motivate me. I posted the collage in a prominent position on my dorm room wall. I cut out a picture of my favorite female fashion model, and pasted a photo of my face on top of hers, hoping that someday maybe I'd really have her body. However, all I was doing was enveloping myself in my weight loss obsession. I wasn't attaining an ideal body, I was just attaining frustration.

*It's estimated that only one percent of women have the genetic makeup to look like the average female model, who is 5'11" and 117 pounds. What is the "ideal" body type you are striving for? Is it realistic for you? How has your ideal been shaped by fashion magazines, billboards, and movie and TV stars?*

## THE QUEST FOR SUCCESS

By my junior year in college, weight loss wasn't about pleasing others any more. It had become a matter of principle to me. I just had to succeed at weight loss. *Had to.* I was determined to find some plan, some way to lose weight. I'd be ravenous by lunch, and then would typically end up snacking the rest of the day and evening. I tried weight loss centers, but couldn't stand the regimented meal plans. I tried diet shakes as meal replacements, which never satisfied my hunger so I'd often end up having the shake *plus* regular food. I noticed that I tended to binge when I ate sugar, so I tried cutting out sugar completely. After several months of being sugar-free, I couldn't stand the deprivation so I let myself have sugar, but only once a week. Of course, this turned into an all-out sugar binge on that one day each week. The more weight loss games I played, the more frustrated I felt. It seemed as if no matter what I tried, I could not succeed. The more I focused on weight loss, the worse my weight problem became. But I wasn't going to give up!

*If you've tried losing weight for any length of time, you have probably encountered many failures. Has this made you even more determined to succeed? What have you been willing to do in order to succeed? What's the most drastic thing you've ever done to lose weight?*

## THE QUEST FOR WILLPOWER

After finishing my fourth and final year as a varsity athlete, I shifted to an apathetic extreme, rebelling against exercise since I felt I had been forced to do it for so long. I also abandoned my diet rules, adopting an "I don't care" attitude. I was just tired of trying so hard. I felt out of control with food, often finding it hard to stop eating once I started. *My weight problem had turned into apathy, and I began to develop another type of eating disorder called binge eating.* Binge Eating Disorder is characterized by recurrent episodes of compulsive overeating. But as my weight quickly ballooned, reaching 175 pounds on my 5'6" frame, I started to panic. From apathy I shifted back to rigidity, digging deep inside myself for all the willpower I could find. I weighed myself every morning and recorded my weight. I wrote everything I ate in a food diary, and calculated every calorie I burned. If I ate what I judged to be an acceptable amount, and if I burned an adequate number of calories, then I gave myself a pat on the back. If I slipped from the plan, I analyzed what I needed to do differently and vowed to implement it. With this rigid control I did finally start to lose weight, but all my thoughts revolved around weight control. I thought about what I should eat, when I should exercise, how long to exercise to burn off what I'd eaten, and I kept a running tally of calories in my head all day long. The margins of my college class notebooks were filled with my calorie counts. I was more interested in weight loss than in my studies. Controlling my weight had become my life's purpose, and reaching my goal weight was the most important goal in my life.

*What is your willpower like right now? How do you think your willpower is related to your ability to control your weight?*

## THE QUEST TO HAVE YOUR CAKE AND EAT IT TOO

I had only so much willpower. Like Dr. Jekyll and Mr. Hyde, it didn't take much to turn me from a rigidly disciplined dieter to a ravenous monster, eating everything in sight. One day, feeling disgusted with myself after eating so much, I decided to try a "weight loss secret" that one of my high school girlfriends had shared with me. She made herself throw up after eating, and she said this allowed her to eat whatever she wanted without getting fat. At first, I used this "secret" only if I felt I had eaten too much, perhaps once a week. But then it became a crutch, a way for me to "have my cake and eat it too," a way to eat what I wanted but not suffer the weight consequences of it. I began to purge several times a week, then once a day, then several times a day. Then I started buying any food I liked, knowing I could just gorge myself and then throw up. Any time I felt pressure in relationships, school, work, or family life, I numbed the pain with my binges and purges. *My weight problem had turned to obsession and evolved into bulimia.* Bulimia Nervosa is an eating disorder characterized by compulsive phases of binge eating followed by purging; a purge is any method used to "get rid of" what has been eaten, such as self-induced vomiting, laxatives, diuretics. Fasting or exercising to compensate for calories consumed in a binge are also considered bulimic behaviors.

*Have you ever wished you could eat everything you wanted and still lose weight? Have you ever overdone it with your eating, then purged to compensate? What methods have you used to purge, or "get rid of," what you have eaten?*

## THE QUEST TO BE GOOD ENOUGH

Besides getting thin, part of my master plan had been to meet a man in college and get married. But it didn't happen. In fact, I never even had a serious boyfriend. I had pretty much concluded I wasn't "good enough" for any man. So I had to modify this master plan and move on with my life without that husband. Under much influence from my family and peers, I decided to pursue a career as a bioengineer. The summer before my graduate program started, I finally met a man who actually seemed to think I was good enough after all! But just as I started to believe that he really liked me, I found out that he was still spending time with his old girlfriend. If I really was good enough, why was he spending so much time with her? I discovered how thin his ex-girlfriend was, and I was convinced that I had to be as thin as her if I was to hold onto him. I associated "good enough" with "thin enough." Even though he never intimated that I should lose weight, I concluded that this was how he felt. I thought I was lucky to have this new boyfriend, and I just *knew* he'd break up with me if I didn't get my body trimmed down *fast*. This fueled my eating disorder, and my bulimia symptoms worsened as I binged and purged several times each day.

*How have your relationships with "significant others" influenced your weight loss behaviors? What kinds of messages have you learned from your significant others, either directly or indirectly? What conclusions have you made about being "good enough"?*

## THE QUEST TO BE PERFECT

I felt extreme pressure to please others in graduate school. When I had my first meeting with my advisor, he informed me that I had just made the cutoff to get into the program. He told me how challenging my classes and research would be, and he indicated that I needed to prove myself to him. He said, "I expect you to get A's." I felt as if I had been thrown into icy cold water without being taught how to swim. Some say this is the rite of passage in graduate school, a test to see if you will sink or swim. Determined to swim, I did everything I could to make my way through this new territory. I never let my advisor know how confused or overwhelmed I felt. I did everything I could to appear perfect; and, to cope with my fear that he wouldn't approve of me, I returned to my eating disorder. I engaged in a combination of restrictive eating and purging, in which I would often throw up what little I did eat and then exercise to burn off any calories that might have "gotten through." My weight dropped to 120 pounds, which was thin for my 5'6" muscular frame. But I didn't see myself as thin—I still wanted to lose more weight. *My extreme drive to lose weight even though I was already thin was a sign that I was becoming anorexic all over again.*

*Have you ever been faced with demands or expectations from someone, but felt unable to meet them? Have you been in other situations where you felt pressure to please someone? How has controlling your weight been your way to be perfect?*

## THE QUEST FOR HAPPINESS

The more I focused on losing weight, the heavier it weighed upon my soul. My core essence was buried beneath all my weight loss games. The fact that my soul was being weighed down didn't concern me, because I was convinced that I was flawed at my core. I was convinced that my inner guidance would lead only to humiliation and failure. I was convinced that the key to happiness was to be found *outside* myself. After fifteen years I had come full circle—from my lowest weight as an anorexic young girl to my highest weight, bordering on obesity, as an adult, and then losing weight almost to the point of anorexia all over again. I had searched the world over, tried every weight loss game I could find or devise, and yet during that entire time *I never found the answer.*

*Where have you been looking for happiness? Have you tried losing weight as a means to finding happiness? How has weight control influenced your happiness over the years? What are some of your other reasons for trying to lose weight? Have you found what you are questing for, or are you still searching? Where do you think you will find what you're seeking?*

# the games
# dieters play

I finally solved my food, weight, and body worries, and went on to specialize in the field of assisting others with weight problems and eating disorders. Today, I don't know my exact weight because I step on the scale only at my doctor's office for my yearly checkup. At 5'6" tall, I comfortably wear a size 6, and I estimate that I weigh approximately 130 pounds. More important than how much I *weigh* is how I *feel*—happy, healthy, balanced, peaceful, and confident. I achieved and now maintain my present status *without* diets or other weight loss games. But before I tell you how I overcame my struggles and how I guide others to do the same, I want to tell you more about the games people play to lose weight and *why none of them work*. We create the games, and we also create the rules. But we set up the games and the rules so that we can't possibly win. Let's look at some of the games.

## The Magic Pill Game

There are pills that claim to decrease appetite, speed up metabolism, prevent fat from being stored, or even melt the excess fat from your body. If only, if only, *if only* it were true! Well, it might be. Better try it and find out. After all, there's a 30-day money-back guarantee; what could it hurt to try? One problem with pills is that they *all* have side effects. None of the pills are designed for long-term use. Also, many of the pills promote weight loss through depletion of water from the body. Sometimes pills can have such a diuretic (water-losing) effect that dehydration or kidney failure can result. Even "natural" or "herbal" pills are not healthy. The major problem with any pill is that if weight loss does occur, it is only because the pill addressed the *symptom*. No changes were made in the behaviors that brought about the initial weight gain, so once the pills are stopped, the weight comes back.

## The Diet Game

This game has many different names, depending on the type of diet. The basic concept, though, is to rigidly adhere to a specific meal plan or set of food requirements for the day. Often, the game requires eating only at specific times of day. The diet game can result in weight loss—*if* you stick to it long enough. However, once you go off the diet and return to your old eating habits, you will regain the lost weight. Diets do not result in lasting success and freedom from weight problems; they are only temporary solutions that often backfire. Because metabolism often slows down during periods of restrictive eating, as during dieting, it is common to eventually gain back the lost weight—and usually more.

## THE CALORIE COUNTER GAME

While it might seem logical that eating fewer calories will result in weight loss, the reality is that dramatically cutting calories results in a loss of lean tissue (muscle) rather than fat. Weight loss will occur, but it's due to the loss of muscle, which in turn lowers metabolism. That's why, after the calorie counting stops, it can be so easy to regain the lost weight. Calorie counting can become an obsession; thoughts are often focused on the daily tally sheet—how many calories have been eaten, and how many are still "allowed"? But why spend all that mental energy counting calories? Aren't there better things to think about?

## THE FAT GRAM GAME

Fewer than 30 grams of fat a day. No, better make it fewer than 20. No, fewer than 10. People who play this game can spend hours reading nutrition labels. They usually won't eat something unless they can see the label and calculate the fat grams. If the serving has more than two grams of fat, forget it. Fat-free is the goal. They'll dine out, but only if they can order from a menu that lists the fat grams in each dish. What a lot of effort! Unfortunately, playing this game has many negative consequences. First, fat in the diet plays an important role in satiety (feeling full), so the person who is severely restricting fat will always feel hungry and will always be thinking about food and eating. She will often spend all her spare time planning the next meal, sometimes planning days ahead. Second, fat in the diet is essential for our bodies to properly absorb the fat-soluble vitamins A, E, D, and K. You can watch the pounds come off, and watch your hair fall out too, as a result of nutrient deprivation.

## The Good-Food Game

Here the idea is to eat only "good" foods and to cut out anything considered a "bad" food. Typically, "good" foods include fruits, vegetables, grains, legumes, and anything else low in fat. "Bad" foods include cakes, cookies, candy, sugar, fried foods, high-fat dairy, and most meats. The problem is that, psychologically, we always want what we can't have. The minute you say to yourself, "I won't eat any of that chocolate cake," you will find that you can't stop thinking about it. Eventually, this game backfires and can lead to an all-out binge on the so-called bad foods. Also, this game can result in insufficient fat intake. Besides feeling hungry all the time, you may also suffer the consequences of being deprived of the fat-soluble vitamins, which cannot be utilized by the body without enough dietary fat.

## The Granola Bar Game

Think of a food that makes you feel satisfied, but that you can't overeat. Then, eat only that food. Take granola bars, for instance. Maybe you could eat four or even six at a time, but there's no way you'd ever want more. So, eat only granola bars for breakfast, lunch, and dinner. If you limit yourself to only this one food, then you will never overeat. However, with such a restrictive diet it is impossible to provide the body with all the nutrients it needs. You can watch the pounds come off, and also notice poor skin quality and other complications brought on by nutrient deprivation.

## The Healthy Eater Game

This game starts out with good intentions. But, what begins as an attempt to be healthy can often lead to overly restrictive eating. In general, this game involves following the U.S. RDA (Recommended Daily Allowance) guidelines, and using the food pyramid to structure eating. These are truly healthy guidelines, designed to maximize health and minimize the risk of certain diseases. The problem occurs when people become overly rigid about the guidelines, or start to change the guidelines, thinking "more of this and less of that will be better." Often, people misinterpret the guidelines. The best example of misinterpretation is with the guidelines for fat consumption. People read the guideline that 30 percent of total calories should come from fat, and then think that means to eat less than thirty grams of fat per day. Actually, 30 percent of total calories for the average female translates to about 75 grams of fat, and for the average male, about 90 grams of fat. This game is also overly focused on the external guideline of "What should I eat?" versus the internal guideline of "What does my body need to function at its best?"

## THE SIX-ON, ONE-OFF GAME

For the first six days, you need to be "on plan," which typically means low-fat, low-calorie, no desserts, and so on. Then, on the seventh day, you can go "off plan" and have anything you want. Sounds pretty good, until you end up in an all-out binge every week on the seventh day, or when you finally can't stand to "be good" for six days in a row so you start giving yourself two off-days, then three, then four, then . . .

## THE 6:00 P.M. GAME

Never, never, never eat after 6:00 P.M. Everything you eat after this point will turn to fat. Hmm, that's a mystery, because our bodies need fuel twenty-four hours a day, even when we sleep. Whoever started this game didn't have all the facts. If you are hungry after 6:00 P.M. but *don't* eat, your metabolism will slow down, you won't sleep well, and you'll be wanting *more* food the next day.

## THE FASTING GAME

This game involves fasting for one, two, or more days each week. Sometimes the game is a liquid fast; at other times, even liquids are eliminated. The body is an amazing thing: It has preservation mechanisms to keep itself alive during times of famine. However, these preservation mechanisms were not intended for weight loss! Fasting is very hard on the body, and if liquids are restricted, severe dehydration can result. You might temporarily lose weight, but you will rapidly regain it when you start to eat again.

## THE JUMP-START GAME

Here the goal is to lose weight *fast*, to get that "jump start" and then focus on maintaining your new, lower weight. Many people want something to motivate them, something to feel good about; seeing that number on the scale go down can be a positive reinforcer to stick to the game. However, if the number drops more than two pounds a week, the weight loss is mostly water or muscle. Water weight will be regained when the "jump-start" phase is over. The loss of muscle will result in a slowing of the metabolism, making it easier to regain the lost weight—plus a few extra pounds. Another problem with this game is that the follow-up "maintenance plan" is just another diet that is impossible to adhere to. So you'll go back to your old patterns and gain weight back even *faster* than you lost it.

## THE WATER GAME

In this game, the idea is to drink lots of water, especially before meals, to feel fuller. Although you may feel fuller for a while, the water will rapidly move out from your stomach and on to your kidneys, and you'll go back to being hungry—possibly *too* hungry, which can trigger a binge. Another concept of this game is that drinking lots of water can "flush out" body fat. Our bodies do need water, but excess amounts of it will only result in more frequent urination. It is not possible to "flush out" fat!

## THE SCALE GAME

With this game, you rely upon the scale to determine your eating and activity for the day. If you have gained since your last weigh-in, you have to watch your food intake and try to skip meals; in addition, you have to exercise more so that you can lose whatever you gained. If you stay the same, you also have to watch your food intake and exercise more so that you can lose. If you lose, you still have to watch your food intake and exercise more so that you can lose *more*. No matter what the scale says, you can't win.

## THE EXERCISE GAME

Everyone knows that exercise burns calories. So to lose more or to lose faster, why not exercise more? How about two or three hours a day? The more the better. It doesn't matter whether you like to exercise or not, you just have to make yourself do it. Discipline. Hard work. Sweat. That will make the weight come off, or so you think. In reality, pushing yourself this hard adds to your stress level, which can result in an *increased* desire to eat. Also, exercising too hard can have harmful consequences, including injury, dehydration, or chronic fatigue.

## THE NO-CAL BEVERAGE GAME

In this game, all calories count. Why waste calories on beverages? Why not have only no-calorie drinks as a way to cut calories? Think of all the calories that can be saved by having only calorie-free beverages! The problem here is that the calories in beverages do contain nutrients our bodies need. If they are eliminated, it can be difficult to get all the required nutrients. For example, fruit juice and milk both contain calories, but also many necessary vitamins, minerals, and other nutrients. Cutting out calories from beverages will only result in the desire to eat more in order to compensate.

## THE TRADE-OFF GAME

Did you exercise today? If you did, you can eat. The type and duration of exercise will determine the type and amount of food you can eat. Also, if you eat, you then have to exercise to burn off what you ate. A piece of pie means an hour of running. This game takes the "calories in, calories out" formula too seriously. It is true that exercise expends calories and eating increases calorie intake. However, you don't need to exercise every time you eat, or eat only after exercising the right amount. This pattern will lead to frustration and a sense of deprivation, and negative attitudes about food and exercise.

## THE SKIPPING GAME

Skip breakfast—and even better, skip lunch, too—to save on calories. Then have whatever you want for dinner. This game is also played when a festive evening is planned: Skip meals to "save up" for the big party. What usually happens, though, is that your hunger is so great by dinnertime that you overeat. Plus, your metabolism slows down in response to your fasting during the day. Meal-skipping cuts calories initially, but almost always results in overeating and weight gain.

## THE HI-PRO GAME

This game involves following a special kind of diet in which carbohydrate foods are reduced or eliminated. Protein and fat may still be consumed. Because the body is not getting enough carbohydrates, glucose cannot be produced to keep the body functioning. Therefore, protein must be converted to glucose. Protein from the diet as well as from the body's own stores (muscle) are thus converted into glucose. Water is a by-product of this conversion, and so the body can lose a substantial amount of water weight. This process can result in weight loss, but mostly due to loss of water and of the body's lean tissue, its muscle. This metabolic process is extremely hard on the kidneys and liver, and will result in weight gain once the diet is discontinued. In addition, the high fat content of this diet can lead to heart disease. Our bodies are just *not* designed to function on low or no carbohydrates!

## THE COMBO GAME

This game requires that you eat special food combinations to speed up metabolism and burn excess fat from your body. The combinations must be followed exactly as written, with no substitutions. It doesn't matter how strange the combinations may sound. A hardboiled egg served with prune juice. A baked potato sprinkled with cayenne pepper. A can of tuna consumed with a grapefruit. You may lose weight doing this, but not because the food combinations are anything special. Rather, it is probably because the combinations are so unappetizing that you don't want much, or because the portion sizes are controlled so you eat less. Once you stop the food combinations, you will regain the lost weight. And who can eat those combinations forever? Is that any way to live?

## THE FOOD DIARY GAME

Here, you must write down everything you eat. You must try, of course, to eat only "good" foods. If you eat something "bad," then you must berate yourself for doing it so it won't happen again. However, all that happens is that you get depressed because you can't seem to stick to your diet. You put yourself down for not having enough motivation. Then, because you feel so down about yourself, you'll probably head to the cupboard for something to eat because you figure you already "blew it."

## THE FAT & UGLY GAME, VERSION I

This one involves eating in your underwear, or even naked, so that you can see how fat and ugly you really are. The thought is that once you see yourself this way, you won't want to eat. Unfortunately, viewing yourself as fat and ugly results in feelings of depression, shame, guilt, and hopelessness, with a lessened desire to take care of yourself. It can seem like weight loss will never happen. Thus you are likely to find yourself wanting to overeat for comfort.

## THE FAT & UGLY GAME, VERSION II

This version involves obtaining photos of obese people and pasting them on the refrigerator, and/or placing a toy pig in the fridge that is programmed to "oink" when the door is opened. This game belittles people who are obese, and also creates feelings of shame and guilt associated with eating. As with Version I, the usual outcome is to overeat, and of course to want to trample on that little pig!

## THE SKINNY IDEAL GAME

This game is similar to the Fat & Ugly Game, Version II. It involves pasting photos of skinny people all over the refrigerator and in other strategic locations. Going one step further, this game involves finding a photo of the ideal body you'd like for yourself, and then pasting a photo of *your* face onto it. But rather than feeling motivated when you see this self-you-are-not, you'll probably end up frustrated that you aren't there yet. When you do give in and eat, feelings of failure set in. Frustration + failure = lots and lots of cookies.

## THE ALLERGY GAME

Some people have convinced themselves that they are allergic to certain foods, so they will not eat them. Food allergies are real; if you suspect an allergy, get a professional medical opinion. Many people "make up" an allergy because they don't know how else to control their food intake. This type of control is not effective in the long run. You will only feel deprived, and end up overeating *other* foods.

## THE HATE GAME

For this game, you need to convince yourself that you really hate the foods that you think are fattening. While eating these fattening foods, you might watch a gory movie. You then need to associate the gore with the food, so that you feel nauseous. All this game does is make for an unpleasant eating experience, and won't ultimately change your behavior.

## THE SUBLIMINAL GAME

Here, you listen to tape-recorded messages that state over and over how much you enjoy foods like fruits and vegetables, and how much you hate foods like desserts or fried items. The idea is to reprogram the subconscious mind to reject high-fat foods. But the reality is that your conscious mind is onto the game. You will find yourself still wanting these foods, but literally being at war with yourself over having them. You can probably eat well for a while, but eventually you will probably end up bingeing on all those foods you really do love that you've tried to convince yourself to hate.

## THE CLOSET GAME

What better way to make oneself lose weight than to have only clothes that are too small in one's closet! No, not really. All that happens here is that you'll be embarrassed to go out in public because nothing fits. If you do go out, you'll wear sweat pants and a sweat top and hope that you don't see anyone you know. And, while you're out, you'll probably swing by the fast-food drive-thru for something to eat to help you cope with your weight frustration.

## THE NO-TRIGGER GAME

In this game, you identify foods that "trigger" you to overeat and eliminate them from your diet. The problem here is, what if *everything can trigger you to overeat?* Then what do you do? Eliminating foods that you enjoy just because you occasionally eat too much of them will only leave you feeling deprived and frustrated. You will constantly find yourself thinking of all those foods you have told yourself you can't have. Eventually, you may end up in a binge. Wouldn't it make more sense to learn how to eat those foods you enjoy, *without overeating them?*

## THE SURGERY GAME

This game involves various kinds of surgery, from liposuction to stomach stapling, designed to reduce the size of the body or the size of the stomach. However, surgery on the stomach or another body part does not address the reasons *why* you overeat. Many people who have had these surgeries still want to eat the same amount of food as before; they tend to cram the food in, even if the stomach is smaller, and thus they gain weight again.

## THE LIFESTYLE CHANGE GAME

You have probably heard that if you could just develop a "healthy lifestyle" you wouldn't have a weight problem. However, most lifestyle-change programs are actually diets in disguise. Anytime you are given a list of foods to avoid or restrict, be prepared to feel deprived because you can't have them. Similarly, when you are given a rigid exercise plan, you will likely view exercise as a punishment and find yourself wanting to rebel. When rules are imposed from the outside, it is just a matter of time before you'll abandon them and revert back to your old ways.

## THE BEHAVIOR-MODIFICATION GAME

This game involves developing various strategies designed to increase eating awareness and prevent overeating. For example, you might learn to "eat at table only," meaning that you can eat only while seated at the table. Some such strategies are helpful, but others create obsessive eating patterns that can actually result in overeating. If you should happen to "make a mistake" (for example, eat at the "wrong" place), you will typically feel like a failure and find yourself turning to food as a means to cope.

## THE RICE CAKE GAME

Whenever you feel hungry, have a rice cake. The idea here is that you can fill up on "fat-free" foods so that you'll eat less. But because rice cakes have so little fat, and fat is what helps you to feel full, it will actually take *a lot* of rice cakes for you to feel satisfied. If all you eat is rice cakes, you will become severely nutrient-deprived. If you consume rice cakes in addition to other foods, you may find that you eat more calories than you realize. Even though rice cakes are called "fat-free," they are not calorie-free. If you eat rice cakes just to "fill up" but you really want another type of food instead, be prepared to overeat the rice cakes and then probably give in later to have what you really wanted, too.

## THE CABBAGE SOUP GAME

This game involves following a specific diet that includes, of course, cabbage soup. People have been known to experience diarrhea playing this game, and any weight loss that occurs is probably due to water loss. Just like other diets, when you go back to your regular eating patterns, you can expect to regain all the weight you lost.

## THE SMOKING GAME

Many people take up smoking because they think it will speed up their metabolism and thus promote weight loss. If nicotine has any such effect on metabolism, the benefit is not worth the substantial risk of disease that smoking presents. Developing lung cancer in an attempt to be thin is *truly* not worth it!

## THE CAFFEINE GAME

Load up on black coffee, diet cola, and anything else with caffeine. It's often thought that caffeine, like nicotine, can rev up the metabolism. While caffeine does not pose the health risks that smoking cigarettes does, high doses will not promote long-term weight loss. You will probably just find yourself experiencing headaches and irritability. There is no substance that you can ingest as a "magic cure" for a weight problem.

## THE CHEWING GUM GAME

Pop a piece of gum (sugarless, of course) into your mouth whenever you feel hungry. When you are chewing gum, you can't eat. Be prepared to go through packs and packs of gum each day, and also be prepared to binge when you finally do let yourself eat. When your body signals you that you need to eat, chewing gum will not provide the nutrients you need. Ignoring your hunger cues will only backfire in the end.

## THE NAIL POLISH GAME

Put fresh nail polish on your nails to prevent yourself from eating at key times; for example, during the evening. You'll eat less, and have great nails, too! However, will you really eat less? If your body needs food and you ignore the signals, you will probably overeat at the next meal. Also, any time you don't eat when you are truly hungry you set yourself up for a slowed metabolism.

## THE BARE KITCHEN GAME

Eliminate from your home all foods that you might overeat. Fill your fridge and cupboards with only "good" foods. However, even if you have only "good" foods around, you can still overeat. A calorie is a calorie, whether it's in a carrot or a cookie. Unless you get in touch with what drives you to overeat, you will probably still find yourself eating more "good" food than your body needs. In addition, if you have eliminated all the foods you really enjoy because you are concerned that you will overeat, then you will set yourself up for a deprivation-induced binge.

## THE DIET TOMORROW GAME

This is a popular game that is played while on vacations or during the holidays. In this game, you give yourself permission to completely overindulge in all the foods you love, knowing that you will start a restrictive eating plan soon. You allow yourself to eat all the foods you enjoy, just to say "good-bye" before your period of fasting. You will gorge today, then diet tomorrow . . . or maybe put off the diet until the next day . . . or the next day . . .

## THE WEDDING GAME

Do you have a special occasion coming up? Perhaps a wedding, a reunion, or a cruise? Then you'd better get the weight off *fast!* Special events can often serve as the initial motivation to begin a diet. However, if you lose pounds for a special occasion, be prepared to gain the weight back after the event is over. Once the motivation is gone, you'll revert back to your old patterns.

## THE SWEAT GAME

Desperate for weight loss? The body is made up of more than 65 percent water. Why not lose some water weight by sweating? Try a sauna, or wearing a rubber suit while exercising, to make you lose water through sweating. Diuretics (water pills) also force the body to lose water. This type of weight loss game is extremely dangerous, and can be fatal. The body has a delicate balance of its fluids, and dehydration can quickly result in *death*. Is it worth it to be thin, if it means being thin in your coffin?

## The Purging Game

Want to "have your cake and eat it too"? If you eat a meal and then regurgitate, this can reduce the full feeling you have after eating, and can also reduce the calories absorbed by the body. Taking laxatives has a similar effect. However, if you play this game regularly, you probably have an eating disorder. Purging puts you at high risk for rupturing your esophagus, having major gastrointestinal complications, experiencing nutrient deficiency, and going into heart failure due to electrolyte imbalance.

*Take some time and reflect upon the various games you have played to try to reach your weight loss goals. How have the games worked? Have the games you played provided a lasting solution, or merely a "quick fix"? Which games have actually posed a health risk? Have you been able to win the weight loss games? If not, what do you think has been stopping you? How can you have the success you desire?*

# lighten your load

## by losing the games

A half-eaten carton of ice cream, the leftover crusts from an entire deep-dish pizza, an empty box of pop-tarts, a portion of a two-liter bottle of diet soda, a few cookies, and crumbs all over the coffee table, couch, and floor. This is all that remains as I continue with my hour-long binge and purge ritual. It's a familiar routine. I eat so much that I can barely walk to the kitchen, where I lean over the sink and put my right index finger down my throat, forcing myself to throw up just enough food so that I can go back and eat more. "What are ya doin'?" asks Peppy, my parakeet, as I shove more cookies and ice cream into my mouth. "Shut up!" I scream back at him. Until finally I can't stand the thought of stuffing down anything else.

Now it's time to vomit until I get everything out. *Get rid of it all.* I drink more diet soda to make the vomiting easier. I throw up as much as I can, praying that my esophagus doesn't rupture in the process. *Shouldn't have eaten that pizza, too hard to throw up.* I drink more diet soda and throw up again, and again, and again. "What are ya doin'?" asks Peppy again. *Stupid bird.* I drink more diet soda, then throw up several more times. *Damn. No pop-tarts yet.* I always eat cherry pop-tarts first when I binge, and they're always the last to come back up. When I see the pop-tarts, then I know I'm almost done. I drink more diet soda, then throw up again in a few more forceful bursts. *Yes! Pop-tarts, there they are! Now get them all out.* When only the diet soda comes back up, when there is no trace left of any food, then and only then will I stop.

Exhausted, I pause for just an instant to catch my breath, clinging to the kitchen sink. "What are ya doin'?" Peppy says as he flies over to me, landing on my shoulder. "Go away," I retort, as I agitatedly brush him off my shoulder. *Almost there. Just one more time.* I drink more diet soda, and engage in one final purge. Finally, only diet soda is coming up. I can stop. I run the disposal and wash away all the traces of vomit. Disgusted, I glance over at the coffee table and grab the carton of ice cream and remaining cookies. I dump the leftover food down the disposal. *This is the last time.* But that's what I always say. I head into the bathroom, where I catch a glimpse of a red-faced, teary-eyed, puffy-cheeked woman in the mirror, and I wonder who she is. I look away. I wash the vomit off my face, and rinse my mouth out with mouthwash. I drink a small amount of watered-down juice and take a vitamin. I clean up the crumbs, wrappers, boxes, and food remnants from the coffee table. "What are ya doin'?" Peppy asks again. *I don't want to think about it.* I leave no trace of the part of me that feels so out of control.

I go back into the bathroom and gingerly step on the scale,

watching with anxious anticipation as the needle steadies on the number that reflects my weight . . . the number that reflects my life . . . 122 pounds. *Damn. Up half a pound.* Disciplined, I put on my running clothes, preparing to head out for my ten-mile run. *I've got to burn off any calories that may have gotten through.* "What are ya doin'?" Peppy repeats. I pause. Suddenly I see everything that I have just done in a flash. I clearly see the pattern that I repeat every day, often several times a day. Finally I am able to see the insanity of it all. *Peppy's right. What am I doing?*

## WAKING UP FROM THE DIET NIGHTMARE

You've probably heard the adage, "Insanity is doing the same thing over and over, but expecting different results." So is that why I lived a diet nightmare for more than fifteen years? Is that why I kept looking for the latest and greatest method to solve my weight problem? Is that why I was willing to risk my life? Truly, this was insanity.

Sadly, I am not alone in this experience. Just as I began my first diet at age ten, recent studies reveal that two-thirds of American girls have already been on their first diet by their tenth birthday. It's estimated that 100 million Americans are trying to lose weight on any given day. Of these, 35 percent are considered to be overly obsessed with weight control, showing various symptoms of eating disorders. Approximately 10 million Americans are currently in treatment for Anorexia Nervosa and Bulimia Nervosa, with millions more suffering from Binge Eating Disorder and other undiagnosed eating disorders. One recent study indicates that 50 percent of women on American college campuses have eating disorders or are disordered eaters (demonstrating eating disorder symptoms, such as restrictive eating or binge-and-purge patterns, but not severe enough to meet the diagnostic criteria for an eating disorder).

At the other extreme, it's estimated that 55 percent of the American population is overweight or obese. Because chronic dieting can slow the body's metabolism, 90 percent of dieters regain any weight they may lose, and 95 percent end up weighing more than when they started their diet. We are literally dieting our way up to obesity, and obsessing our way down to anorexia. What will it take for us to approach weight loss in an entirely new way, in which both eating disorders *and* obesity can be resolved and ultimately prevented? *What will it take for you to wake up from your diet nightmare?*

Motivational speaker Les Brown told a story about a dog that was moaning and groaning as he lay on the front porch of his home. A passerby asked the dog's owner why the dog was whining so much, and the owner replied, "Because he's lying on a nail." The passerby said, "Well, why doesn't he get off?" And the owner said, "I guess it doesn't hurt bad enough." I was like that dog, lying on a nail for fifteen years. I guess it finally "hurt bad enough" for me to do things differently. It's often said that in order to make a change, one must "hit bottom." But I never "reached the bottom"—I was able to take an objective look at my weight-obsessed life before I had lost everything. I am grateful for that.

In many ways, Peppy served a significant role in giving me my wake-up call. Many parakeets can talk, but why did he choose to say, "What are ya doin'?" on that particular day? Although it was one of his three standard phrases, it was significant that he said *that* phrase while I was bingeing and purging. That phrase was no coincidence. When I finally chose to pay attention to what he was saying, I was able to realize the insanity of all the weight loss games I'd played for years. It was like a movie flashing through my mind, replaying my entire diet nightmare before my eyes. Finally, I could see what I was doing. And I was ready to wake up from my diet nightmare. *Are you? What are* you *doing?*

The real "weight" that I needed to lose was the burden of my diet nightmare. My "weighty attitudes" were what had been feeling so heavy. It's like I was carrying around a big canvas bag full of all of my dieter's games. It was my "dieter's bag of tricks," and each time I tried a new weight loss strategy, I added it to my bag. However, the more I tried to lose weight, the more that weight loss eluded me. *The real problem was that I could never seem to be free of my weight problem.* Even if I did lose weight, then I had to worry about how to maintain my weight. This kept me playing more dieter's games, year after year. But after fifteen years, my dieter's bag of tricks was extremely heavy. It had become my "dieter's bag of burdens." I was so worried about how much my body weighed that I didn't even realize the extra mental and emotional "weight" I was carrying. My life revolved around weight control, and I had lost my soul in the process.

What exactly do I mean by the word "soul"? *Webster's Dictionary* defines soul as "the principle of life, feeling, thought, and action in humans, thought of as something distinct or separate from the body; the spiritual part of humans." When I ask people in my workshops to define soul, they give me answers like "connection to the divine," "eternal essence," "True Self," "spirit," and "answers that come from within." You probably have your own sense of what your soul is, and I encourage you to deepen your awareness, understanding, and experience of your soul.

When I use the word *soul,* I consider it to mean the core essence of who we are. With all of my focus on weight control, I had lost connection with my core essence. I didn't know who I was any more, aside from a number on a bathroom scale. My soul was squashed underneath that scale, buried amidst the diet books on my bookshelf, hidden in my closet with those too-tight clothes, crumbled into pieces with the cookies from my binges, and washed down the drain with my purges. *I was so worried about how much my body weighed, but how much did my soul weigh?* My soul felt extremely heavy, just like that "bag of burdens." Perhaps this was my real weight problem—maybe I needed to free myself of the "weight" that was burdening my soul. *How heavy is your "bag of burdens"? How much does your soul weigh?* (To get an estimate, take the Self-Test in Appendix I.)

## DISCOVERING THE REAL "MAGIC PILL"

As a bioengineering graduate student at The University of Michigan, I did research on muscle and bone physiology, and my doctoral dissertation involved osteoporosis treatment and prevention. Based on my experience, an ideal job for me would have been to work at a pharmaceutical company, to assist with the evaluation of new osteoporosis therapies. Women's health issues were of interest to me, and so this would have been a meaningful endeavor. However, the health issue that was still the most important to me was weight loss. The research that I really wanted to do at that pharmaceutical company was to discover the "magic pill"—the one that would solve people's weight problems . . . *forever.*

I didn't realize that I would go on to discover the real magic pill—but that it was not a pill to be developed by a pharmaceutical company and then sold in a bottle. *The real magic pill is something that is already inside of us—it's our intuition, the voice of our soul.* I consider the soul's voice to be a direct communication link with the Higher Power, the Universal Intelligence, or however you may view God. It's like having God's voice within you. If God is the ocean, your soul is a cup of sea water. That cupful contains the same "stuff" that the whole ocean does, just on a smaller scale. Each one of us contains a cupful of God, which is the core essence of our soul. Together, our souls make up the ocean. This vast ocean contains all knowledge, and so does the cupful within you. In her book *Divine Intuition,* Lynn A. Robinson says, "Whatever your belief is about the source, you have access to a deep wisdom that resides in your soul." We can access this wisdom through the soul's voice—our intuition. But it's up to us to listen to the often subtle ways in which our intuition surfaces. *Intuition is your spiritual birthright. Reclaim it.*

*Webster's Dictionary* defines intuition as "direct perception of, or the power of understanding, a fact, the truth, a conclusion, etc., without any reasoning process or analysis." Intuition is an *inner knowing.* Intuition may also be called our inner wisdom, sixth sense, a hunch or gut feeling. You have probably experienced the guidance of your intuition—for example, while driving on the expressway you feel an overwhelming sense that you ought to exit, then find out later that by so doing you avoided an accident or an awful traffic jam. You have probably experienced the negative consequences of *not* honoring your intuition—for example, ignoring the prompting from within to make a commitment to something, only to realize later that you missed an incredible opportunity.

Your intuition is available to help guide you in your daily life. This includes your eating, exercise, and weight issues. But you've probably been trained to discount this valuable source of inherent wisdom. We are all born with intuition, but many of us have forgotten it's there and so we don't listen to it on a regular basis. Our society values logic, facts, proof—all of which stifle intuition. However, you can regain and enhance your intuitive ability. Reclaiming your intuition is the real "magic pill." It offers a holistic solution to weight problems because it addresses the whole person—soul, mind, *and* body—and deals with the cause of weight problems, not just the symptom of weight. *Your real "magic pill" of intuition is within you, and when you learn to listen to it again, your weight problem will solve itself.*

In the following pages I'll tell you how I discovered the real magic pill within myself, and give you the background on how I reconnected with my intuition and how this helped me to solve my own weight problem. Drawing on what I learned to create my own success, I developed the process to help others find the real magic pill within themselves. I have gone before you into uncharted territory, and will provide you with a road map to make your way more clear. But before I give you your map, it will be helpful for you to learn more about how and why the map was developed, based on my own experiences in that uncharted territory. This will enhance your trust in the process, which is essential for your success. My voyage progressed in three steps: body to mind, mind to soul, and soul to freedom. Let's look at what I discovered at each step.

## From the Body to the Mind

By the time I was completing my doctorate in bioengineering, I had taken advanced coursework in physiology, biochemistry, and nutrition, which provided me with a thorough understanding of the basic science of the human body. This knowledge should have been sufficient to give me the ultimate solution to my weight problem. But somehow the science was not enough. At its most basic level, the weight loss formula is very simple: Burn more calories than you take in, and you'll lose weight. Theoretically the formula makes sense, and if it is followed you should lose weight. *But we are more than just a body.* The weight loss formula is impossible to apply and maintain because it ignores the deeper levels of who we are. As a bioengineer, I placed all the emphasis of my research on the body and quantifying physiological processes—the psychological processes were not considered. I had been doing the same with weight control, putting all my focus on the body, trying to control my weight by controlling diet and exercise. But then I thought about the whole concept of control. I concluded that in order to control the body, I needed to control the mind.

So I set out to learn more about the psychology of weight control, and how the mind could assist me in reaching my weight loss goals. I knew that the answer lay beyond standard diets, so I began to look for "don't diet" books. Each week, I visited my favorite bookstore and scanned the weight loss section for new arrivals. At first I was incredibly excited, as I discovered several books that discussed the power of the mind in creating weight loss success. Discipline. Motivation. Willpower. I just needed to train my mind to develop these qualities. I learned about "tummy hunger" (when the body really needs food) versus "head hunger" (when we just want to eat but are not really hungry), and the recommendation was to eat only when hungry. *Eat only when hungry.* This message played in my mind constantly. I wrote it on notecards that I carried around with me. I was determined to develop the discipline to eat only when hungry. This seemed to be the key: mind control for weight control. But then an experience at a birthday party changed my perspective.

I was having a pretty good time at the party, until the cake was served. As it was being passed around, I passed up piece after piece because I heard that message playing in my mind: *Eat only when hungry.* Well, I was not hungry. So, no cake for me. Of course, it was my favorite kind of cake, fudge ripple with chocolate frosting. My friends enjoyed every delectable bite of their cake as I stood by and drooled. One of my slim friends asked, "Aren't you going to have some?" I smiled and said, "No, I'm not really hungry, thanks." But all the while I was thinking how unfair it was that they could have cake and I couldn't. Especially my naturally thin friends—I wondered, How could they eat cake and stay so slim? And with every plate that I touched and then handed to someone else, I could feel deprivation kicking in. I told myself, "Once I'm thin like them, then I can have cake at parties again." But somehow this still didn't resolve the fact that I really wanted cake at that moment, not at some unknown time when I would be thin enough.

Then I had the brilliant idea to take a piece of cake home with me, to eat later when I was actually hungry. I was leaving the party, with my piece of cake wrapped up in a napkin, when it hit me: *I want to have my cake and eat it too.* As a bulimic, that would have meant eating my cake and then throwing it up. But I didn't want that. I wanted to *enjoy eating my cake* just because I wanted a piece, free of guilt or worries about weight gain. I realized that everyone else at the party got to have a piece of cake— were they all hungry, or were they eating cake just because they wanted to? I realized that perhaps the power of the mind was not the answer after all. I thought about all my naturally thin friends. They got to have their cake and eat it too. They could eat cake, even if they were not hungry, and they stayed thin. I wondered, What if I started living like them? If I acted like a naturally thin person, would I end up *being* naturally thin, too? I had been trying to *control* my mind, but perhaps I just needed to *change it. Instead of trying to lose weight, I decided to ACT AS IF I was already thin enough.*

## From the Mind to the Soul

Learning the "secrets" of naturally thin people was a major breakthrough for me. Without even realizing it, I had moved from the level of the mind to the level of the soul. What I learned by observing naturally thin people was how to tap into my own intuition again, reconnecting with the voice of my soul. People who have never had weight problems—those who are naturally thin—have never lost touch with their intuition. That's because *naturally thin people have never tried to lose weight.* Naturally thin people have never been on a diet. Diets make us dumb. Diets get us out of touch with our body's natural ability to regulate weight. Naturally thin people became the model for me, helping me learn to let go of the "diet mentality" and tune in to my own inner wisdom about what to eat, how much to eat, when to eat, and when I actually needed something other than food.

I discovered that I ate for emotional reasons a large proportion of the time, and that naturally thin people do this only occasionally. I realized that I needed to separate my eating from my emotions, and self-help books about overcoming emotional eating and the guidance of an eating disorders counselor helped me with this. I learned to identify my feelings and how to express them in healthy ways, rather than using binges to stuff them down or purges to get rid of them. Consequently, my binge/purge patterns began to diminish. In the past I had tried to control my binges or purges, but with limited success. However, by addressing the cause of my binges and purges—unexpressed emotions—I no longer had a need for my eating disorder symptoms.

My therapist had said, "Complete recovery is possible," and that there would come a day when I would live as if I never had an eating disorder. I remember thinking, "God, I hope she's right." I had read so many books about eating disorders that labeled them a "disease" or "illness" and said "there was no cure"; the best that could be hoped for was to "manage the symptoms" and to "cope day-to-day." Not a good prognosis! In contrast, my therapist's perspective about complete recovery was very refreshing. And it was believable, because she was living it. A former anorexic and bulimic herself, she indicated that she lived completely free of her old weight-obsessed thoughts and behaviors. I observed that she was living much like the naturally thin people I knew, trusting her own intuition.

The process of learning to trust my intuition was like learning how to eat all over again. It took a lot of practice to let go of my fifteen-year-old diet mentality patterns, replacing them with my body's own natural eating process. Rather than choosing what I thought I *should* eat because it was "healthy," I learned how to make food selections based on what my body was really hungry for. I discovered that when I ate exactly what my body needed, I was satisfied with less food. Occasionally I overate, especially foods that I had deprived myself of for so long. But rather than berating myself for being a "failure," I viewed overeating as an opportunity to learn for future success. At first my body gained weight in response to my changing eating habits. This was frustrating and scary, but I knew that the only alternative was to go back to living another diet nightmare—not really an alternative at all. I had a strong inner sense that I was on the right path, and that I needed to keep trusting the process as it unfolded. My body size was bigger than I thought it should be, but I also realized that my body was trying to adjust and adapt as it recovered from years of starvation and binges, weight loss and weight gain. I developed a partnership with my body, trusting it completely and knowing that it was in the process of healing. I knew with certainty that my body would eventually reach its own ideal weight, a weight that I would not have to struggle to maintain.

This was a major turning point for me. For years, I had detested my body, viewing it as an enemy. Finally I had reached a place of self-acceptance. Once again, Peppy, my parakeet, played a role in this process. During my time of self-loathing, Peppy would look at his reflection in the little mirror in his cage and say, "I love you, I love you, I love you." Meanwhile, my dialogue with myself in the mirror was, "I hate you, I hate you, I hate you." (That is, if I even paused long enough to glance at myself in the mirror.) Peppy would continue to gaze at the image of himself with adoration, saying, "Gimme a kiss!" as he'd make a kissing gesture in the mirror with his beak. I used to think it was quite narcissistic of him, but then I began to see the message he was sending me. *Love your Self. Love your whole Self.* Having reached a place of self-acceptance, having developed a partnership with my body, I realized that I did indeed love my Self—all except my body. My body was just OK. But to love my Self, I needed to love my whole Self—soul, mind, and body. "I love you, I love you, I love you," I could hear Peppy saying as he looked at himself in the mirror.

And so I decided to follow Peppy's example, and I went into the bedroom and stood in front of my full-length mirror. First I looked at myself, fully clothed. There I stood, at one of my biggest sizes, back up to a size 16. I just tried to look at my body, without judgment. If I became aware of a critical thought, I let it go. Then I felt drawn to repeat this process, *without any clothes on*. There I stood, looking at my body, scanning every aspect. Face. Arms. Breasts. Belly. Hips. Thighs. I could feel the pain of all the years I had hated my body. I could see my body's own unique beauty, as a home for my soul. I could hear my body calling for me to love it. I looked in the mirror and beheld myself with a sense of awe, and said "I love you" as the tears streamed down my face.

The day after I reached this place of freedom, Peppy died. It was as if he knew that his purpose had been served. At first I was angry at Peppy for leaving me just when I had "gotten the message." I felt that I needed his ongoing support as a reminder. But that's when I realized that the best teachers help us find the answers within ourselves. Without Peppy, I had to rely on the voice of my soul, the "teacher" within myself. This was his true gift—the gift of wings—letting my soul take flight, feeling light and free. As I continued to trust my intuition, acting as if I never had a weight problem or eating disorder, my body began to change size, dropping from a size 16 back down to a size 8 over a period of eight months. A size 8 was where my body seemed to want to be, naturally. It was truly an amazing process: I lost weight without even trying. But more important, I overcame my obsessive food, weight, and body worries. *And I reclaimed my life.*

## From the Soul to Freedom

I discovered that my intuition offered me much more than just guidance on how to manage my weight and overcome my eating disorder. My intuitive voice showed me how to live my entire life—how to truly *live* with meaning and fulfillment. I felt as though I had reconnected with the little girl I had been at ten years old, before I began my first diet. I experienced what I call the "circle of the spirit," knowing that I had reclaimed the innocent, creative, vibrant, free nature of my core essence.

I have kept a journal since my senior year in high school, and I reread some of my entries over the years. Amidst all the obsessive chatter about eating, exercise, and weight, I could see the threads of my soul shining through. These were nurturing, encouraging, and inspiring messages about my health, relationships, career—my whole life. I was expressing my deepest desires, hopes, and dreams, painting a beautiful picture of life beyond the number on the bathroom scale. I realized that, indeed, my intuition had been there all along. I just needed to learn how to listen to it again. I needed to quiet the chatter of the "diet mentality" while turning up the volume of my intuitive voice.

At this early point, the whole process of listening to my body for its eating and exercise needs still felt very new. For the next several months, I focused on solidifying the connection I felt with the voice of my soul. I very consciously made eating and exercise soulful experiences. I practiced mindfulness with my eating, expressing gratitude and appreciation for food and really noticing how food energized me. I enjoyed "fitness for my soul," as I went deeply into the experience of being *in* my body as I exercised. Although others may enjoy indoor workouts, I noticed that I felt most alive while doing outdoor activities, such as hiking or cross-country skiing, enjoying a connection with nature and the world around me. I then began to experiment with letting my whole life be a soulful experience, and I incorporated various spiritual practices into my daily life. I continued to read books to help me with the process of enhancing my intuition, concentrating primarily on topics of personal and spiritual growth. I felt the voice of my soul shouting "Yes!" as I read the wisdom expressed by the authors of these books, as if I were reading something I already knew.

Following my intuition used to be something I was consciously aware of *doing*, but now it was becoming my way of *being*. I call this my time of "nourishing my soul," which lasted for about a year. It was as if my soul had been neglected during all my years of weight obsession, and now I was satisfying its hunger. The more I nourished my soul, the more clearly I could hear its wisdom. There were five affirmations that I wrote in my journal each day, that were the essence of the nourishment for my soul: I Love My Self, I Am True To My Self, I Express My Self, I Give To My Self, I Believe In My Self. Practice of these principles guided me to success in my health, relationships, career, finances—all areas of my life.

One of the most significant changes that I experienced was in my career. I was in a period of job transition, knowing that I did not want to stay in bioengineering research, but unsure of what would have true meaning for me. But then I was guided in my life's purpose as the passion of my soul began to surface. I felt an inner yearning to write about my experience of overcoming my eating and weight problems, and to develop a process to guide others in doing the same. I returned to school to earn my master's degree in counseling, and went on to specialize in working with eating and weight issues ranging from anorexia to obesity. Since that time, I continue to nourish my soul in new ways, and I enjoy living free of weight problems. Free of obsession and free of apathy. Free of anorexia and free of obesity. There are still times when I find an old diet rule or eating disorder symptom creeping in. But I don't expect myself to be perfect. I am aware when these situations occur and I learn from them. I remain on my path of happiness, health, balance, peace, and confidence. Now, as an author, professional speaker, and psychotherapist, *I am living my soul's dream.* Quite a contrast from living my diet nightmare!

## LIGHTEN UP!

Using my own success as a model, I have developed a program to teach you how to find the real "magic pill" within yourself. This is the same process that hundreds of my clients have used to overcome their weight problems, ranging from anorexia to obesity. At first, my clients are often surprised by—and distrustful of—the lack of structure. There are no meal plans. There is nothing to count, weigh, or measure. There are no rigid rules. In fact, the only rule is that *there are no rules.* The key to success is to let go of the diet mentality, to lighten your load by losing your dieter's games. When you are willing to let go of your old ways of thinking about weight loss, when you truly become willing to never diet again, then you've taken the first step on your journey of freedom. *Let go of what does not work so that you can experience what will work.*

Your journey of freedom will be unique. I will provide you with a road map to help you navigate through this new territory of tuning in to your intuition, but ultimately you must choose your own path. Your intuition, the voice of your soul, will guide you on your way. But until you can hear your inner voice more clearly, my clients and I will be your guide. Throughout the next four chapters our voices will speak to you, showing you the steps we took to freedom. Then, in the final chapter of the book, you'll learn the "recipes" to help you "feed your hungry soul."

Are you ready to begin your journey of freedom? All you have to do to get started is lose your dieter's-bag-of-burdens. Make the commitment to forget about traditional weight loss approaches, at least for now (you can always pick up your "dieter's-bag-of-burdens" again, if you choose). Are you ready? What have you got to lose? *Now, after leaving your dieter's games behind, how much does your soul weigh?*

# Section II

# Real Results

# intuitive self-care

If the answer to weight problems is not another diet, exercise regimen, meal plan, or weight loss game, what is it?

*It's a process of Intuitive Self-Care.* I believe, and my clients confirm, that we have all the wisdom we need within us: the amount and type of food that the body needs, the amount and type of exercise that the body needs, and the ability to regulate weight without worrying about it. We also have the guidance we need for every other area of our lives. *All* of these answers are within us.

But why do these answers seem so hard to find?

*Because we aren't looking in the right place.* We tend to look outside ourselves for the answers. We look to diets, meal plans, exercise regimens, and other weight loss games. We follow their rigid rules and strict guidelines. But these only block our awareness of our own inner wisdom. If we intend to solve our weight problems, we need to become inner-guided, reconnecting with the voice of our soul—our intuition. We need to act as spiritual beings having a human experience, not human beings having a worldly experience.

Weight problems are not about weight. Eating disorders are not about eating. We need to go beyond the external symptoms to address the internal cause. From anorexia to obesity and everywhere in between, all these symptoms reflect an attachment to the world and detachment from our intuitive guidance. *When we reconnect with our intuitive guidance, weight problems solve themselves.*

## THE WEIGHT-CONSCIOUS "SELF"

To understand how weight problems begin, consider a model of the weight-conscious "self" (Figure 1). In this model, the "self" is a world/mind/body, representing a "human being having a worldly experience." The self is outer-guided, living life from the outside in. The world is the primary focus, with its ideals and standards of health and beauty. Images of perfect bodies that grace the covers of magazines are worshipped, and messages such as "Belly roll and mega thighs defeated at last!" become a life mission. It is a world of competition, where "survival of the fittest" is the name of the game. The mind is aligned with the world, filled with various demands and expectations. Rigid diet and exercise rules become part of the mind's endless list of "shoulds, musts, and oughts." The body reacts to the mind's dictates, but with great resistance. Negative emotions such as depression, anxiety, and frustration are the result, with attempts to "stuff down" these feelings with food or "get rid of" these feelings by starvation. Weight fluctuates in response. Nowhere in this whole scheme does the soul come into play. In fact, as a world/mind/body, the soul is *invisible.* The soul is *starving.* The soul feels heavy, carrying the weight of the world and the burden of the weight loss games.

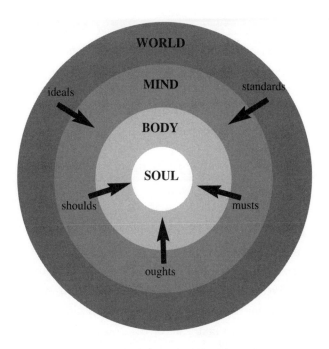

**Figure 1: Model of the "self"**    The "self" is a world/mind/body. The self is outer-guided, looking to the world for its answers. The mind aligns with the world's ideals and standards, and then imposes its demands and expectations on the body in the form of shoulds, musts, and oughts. The soul, while present at the core, is invisible. The soul is starving to be listened to. The overall effect is that the soul feels heavy, carrying the burden of external pressures.

## The Invisible Weight Problem

If you've been living as your weight-conscious "self," caught up in the world's ideals about weight, then you have a weight problem. But no one would know just by looking at you that you have this type of weight problem, because it's *invisible.* This weight problem is *inside* of you, showing symptoms in your mind—what you *think* about your weight. For example, you could be 5'11" and 110 pounds and *still* have a weight problem because you hate your thighs, obsess about food, and constantly worry about maintaining your weight level. Because we can't see thoughts, these weight problems are invisible.

If a person is worried or obsessed about her weight, then she has a weight problem. However, if she is complacent or completely apathetic to weight issues, ignoring her body and her health, she also has a weight problem. This is the classic "I don't care anymore" attitude that can occur after years of living within rigid controls. In the middle is a healthy point of freedom, where one's thoughts are solely about care of the body. No worries, just a healthy regard for the body's needs. No complacency, but yet very little time required to take care of the body. Being free of eating and weight problems means being at the Freedom point in the center of the range of "mental weight" (Figure 2). Note that this continuum ranges from low to high "mental weight"—an avoidance of focus on weight issues (apathy) to extreme weight concerns (obsession).

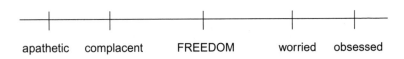

Figure 2. The Range of "Mental Weight"   Weight problems begin in the mind, with what a person thinks about his or her weight. Because thoughts cannot be seen, these are called "invisible weight problems."

Most of you are likely to be to the right of the Freedom point, with weight-worried thoughts some or all of the time. You may be like one of my clients, Sandy, spending every waking moment planning restrictive meals and then dreaming at night about eating hamburgers, French fries, and cake with butter-cream frosting. You are preoccupied with thoughts about your weight, size, or shape, focusing on what it should or shouldn't be. You weigh or measure your body frequently, sometimes multiple times each day. Your mood is usually associated with food, feeling confident or pleased if you eat "good" foods, and feeling anxious or guilty if you eat "bad" foods. You also focus on exercise plans, considering what you should do to burn calories or lose weight. The degree to which these thoughts about weight, eating, or exercise occur determines the severity of your invisible weight problem.

Some of you may fall to the left of the Freedom point, with a lack of concern for eating, exercise, and weight issues. It's often a rebellion against your previous restrictive weight loss methods. It's sometimes an attempt to ignore all the world's ideals because they seem so unattainable. You may be like my client Kristen, giving up on weight control, resigning yourself to being "fat forever." You don't care about your weight, often letting it go to an overweight extreme. You give little regard to food choices, making selections based on whatever costs the least or is most convenient, usually "fast foods." You place minimal focus on exercise, and may be living a completely sedentary lifestyle. The degree to which you block weight, eating, or exercise from your thoughts determines the severity of your invisible weight problem at this extreme.

*Where are you on the mental weight continuum? How much do you think about weight, eating, and exercise, and what has been the result? Can you imagine what a Freedom point would look like, where you'd be free of your "invisible weight problem"?*

## FROM MENTAL WEIGHT TO BODY WEIGHT

External (or body) weight problems—ranging from anorexia to obesity—are the result of invisible (or mental) weight problems. When the mind is out of balance and an invisible weight problem exists, the problem is then transferred to the body as well. The body is pulled from its Freedom point due to worried/obsessive thinking or complacent/apathetic thinking. *Weight problems are manifested when too much focus is placed on weight control.* Weight problems can also occur when the body's health is completely ignored. The lack of balance in both attitudes can cause symptoms such as overeating, binge eating, chronic dieting, or compulsive exercise, which in turn can result in dramatic weight fluctuations. In this sense, anorexia and obesity are flip sides of the same coin.

At the Freedom point, the person's weight is stable and the body is healthy. A natural weight is the weight that the body will achieve on its own, when the mind is free of obsession or apathy. Each person has his or her own healthy, natural weight, which may or may not correspond to an "ideal weight" found on a chart. The natural weight is like a "set point" where the body prefers to be; some people's natural weights will be higher and some will be lower than others'. People may appear to be overweight or underweight according to society's standards, but their bodies may be at the weight that's healthy for them. Being free of eating and weight problems means being at the Freedom point of the range of "body weight" (Figure 3). Note that this continuum ranges from low to high body weight—extremely underweight (anorexia) to extremely overweight (obesity). Also note that low "mental weight" (apathy) can manifest as either low or high body weight (anorexia or obesity), while high mental weight (obsession) can also result in either weight extreme.

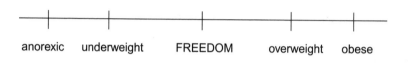

Figure 3. The Range of "Body Weight"   "Visible weight problems" are manifested as the weight problem is transferred from the mind to the body. A person's body weight may be either too high or too low compared to what his or her body weight would naturally be.

Most of you will perceive yourselves to be to the right side of the Freedom point. I say "perceive" because only your body knows the weight that is right for you. You may *think* you are overweight, but this goes back to the invisible weight problem. Observing your weight patterns over time gives an indication of what your natural weight may be. If your weight has fluctuated dramatically, then the Freedom point is probably somewhere in the middle of your lowest and highest weights. The Freedom point is the weight that your body comes back to on its own, when attempts are not being made to control weight. This may be the starting weight before your first diet, or the weight you maintained for brief periods in between diets. Freedom is about trusting your body to take you to the weight that is right for you. At your natural weight, there is no struggle to maintain weight. *This frees you from ever having to play another weight loss game again.*

As your body tries to find its Freedom point, it may respond in a variety of ways. Some people who are overweight will immediately notice a weight loss, while others may notice an initial weight gain before going on to lose weight. This initial weight gain may be due to a slowed metabolism, a common reaction after years of dieting. However, as the body is properly nourished, metabolism tends to correct itself. In the case of the underweight individual, as the body gains weight it may "overshoot" its balanced weight, but then rebound and drop to eventually reach the Freedom point.

At weight extremes, the body can "shut down." In these cases, the anorexic is unable to gain weight and the obese individual is unable to lose weight to get back to the Freedom point, and rigorous intervention may be necessary to reestablish the body's metabolic and other regulatory functions. However, unless you are at an extreme, your body will find its Freedom point on its own. Your body will respond in its own unique way; honor its process.

It may seem difficult at first to let go of the goal of your "ideal" weight. This makes sense, because you've probably had such a weight goal for many years. You have probably convinced yourself that reaching this goal is the key to health and happiness. It's essential to realize that *thinness does not equal health and happiness.* In fact, the quest for weight control compromises both these things. A person who strives to reach her "goal weight" is miserable in the process, living a diet nightmare. Even if she reaches her goal weight, she'll still have her "invisible weight" problem, with a lifetime of worries about how to maintain her thin ideal. The unhealthy extra stress of her weight worries makes her more susceptible to other health complications. In contrast, true health and happiness are an inherent part of the process of reaching the Freedom point of body weight and mental weight. *Health and happiness occur when you lose your weight consciousness.*

*Where are you on the body weight continuum? How has your weight fluctuated over the years? Can you get an idea where your Freedom point is, the weight that's healthy for you that your body can maintain on its own? What's it like to let go of your ideal-weight goal and imagine freedom from your "visible weight problem" in this balanced way?*

## THE SPIRITUALLY CONSCIOUS "SELF"

Solving weight problems requires a shift from a weight-conscious "self" as a world/mind/body to a spiritually conscious "Self" as a soul/mind/body (Figure 4). This model represents a "spiritual being having a human experience." The Self is inner-guided, living life from the inside out. The soul as one's core essence is the primary focus. An intuitive process of Self-care is followed, letting the soul guide the way to the Freedom point of both mental and body weight. The mind is aligned with the soul's wisdom, perceiving it as "intuition," a "sixth sense," or a "gut feeling." The body responds to this inner wisdom with health and balance; the mind becomes free of its "mental weight problem" and the body is freed of its "body weight problem." There is no dependence on the external values of the world. The soul is free of the weight of the world and the burden of weight loss games. There is still interaction with the world, but the purpose of the interaction is to give rather than to get. In this way, the soul is nourished, the mind is enlightened, and the body is at its Freedom point. The Self is whole, healthy, and complete.

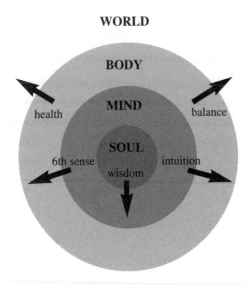

Figure 4: Model of the "Self"   The "Self" is a soul/mind/body. The Self is inner-guided, looking to the soul at its core for answers. The mind aligns with the soul's wisdom, and uses its intuition and sixth sense to guide the body. The body, with health and balance, is then free to interact with the world. The world becomes a place to *give to,* not *get from.* The world is invisible, since the Self is not affected by its influences. The soul is "nourished" as its guidance is listened to. The overall effect is that the soul feels weightless, free of any external pressures.

## THE HEALING OF WEIGHT PROBLEMS . . . AND MORE

We tend to live our lives as the "self," from the outside in. We are outer-guided, seeking answers from the external world. Most of us go through life this way, making our decisions based on advice from outside sources. We live for others' approval, seeking to fit society's ideals. We are convinced that happiness lies in molding ourselves to those ideals. We experience a variety of personal problems, including weight problems, but continue to look outside to the world for answers. However, the more we search for answers, the more elusive the quest. We are merely adding more confusion to our true identity, like placing a mask of "who we think we should be" on top of who we really are. This puts an added burden on our soul, and further separates us from the source of our healing. It is often only when we are carrying such a heavy load from our worldly pursuits that we can realize there must be another way. Sometimes a weight problem (or an alcohol, drug, or other addiction) can be a blessing in disguise. It gets our attention, allowing us to redirect the mind away from the world and back to the soul. In my case, it took fifteen years of struggling and a severe eating disorder to get my attention, but I finally got the message. *Have you?*

My message is to live as the "Self," from the inside out. It is imperative to be inner-guided, to seek answers from the soul. This is how to reconnect with your own process of Intuitive Self-Care. Let your soul guide your mind, and once your mind is in balance, your body will follow. A balanced mind yields a balanced body. If you solve your "mental weight problem" first, your "body weight problem" will take care of itself. Healing begins the moment you choose to align your mind with your soul instead of with the world. Healing will solve weight problems . . . and much more. You will discover a happiness that is independent of the ideals of the world. You will find a peace that goes beyond the circumstances of the world. And you will find a life that is fuller than you ever imagined. You will discover what true freedom from eating disorders and weight problems is all about: the ability to live the life you are meant to live, with your soul nourished, alive and free. *Are you ready to let your soul guide the way?*

*Can you hear your soul's wisdom right now? What is it saying? At first, it may not seem that you are receiving any guidance from within, but this guidance is always there. Reading the upcoming chapters will give you feedback about what others' souls are saying, which can help you tune into your own inner wisdom.*

## MAKING THE TRANSITION

When you first begin the shift from being outer-guided to inner-guided, you may encounter some challenges. Your mind may feel "split," with half wanting to continue its soul-searching and the other half wanting to turn back to the world. The world has a powerful allure, like an elaborate picture frame embedded with jewels: a new diet; a new diet pill; a new weight loss plan. Shiny, bright, and appealing. However, the world offers only empty promises—that elaborate picture frame contains no picture at all. In contrast, your soul offers you a picture more beautiful than any you have ever seen—the image of your core essence. It has a unique beauty in this moment, and yet the artwork is not complete. It is a work in progress, which you add to as your life unfolds. It reflects your entire life experience from the perspective of your soul. This picture has a simple yet sturdy frame that allows your own brilliant work of art to stand out, and symbolizes your being *in* the world, but not *of* the world. So which will you choose—the elaborate empty frame or your real work of art? You won't make this choice just once. Every time you are tempted by what the world seems to offer, you get to choose again. *So what will you choose, the world or your soul?*

As you begin your journey of freedom, it may seem unfamiliar and therefore uncomfortable. It's like opening your front door to find a cold winter day, with the snow blowing and the wind gusting in your face. It would seem much more comfortable to stay right where you are, safe inside your warm, familiar house. To step outside might seem too scary or difficult. How will you survive out in the cold? How will you find your way in a blizzard? What if the storm doesn't let up? What if you leave your comfort zone, only to wish you hadn't? These are all realistic concerns. I have had them, and my clients have as well. The key is to know that the blizzard is only temporary. Knowing this, you can bundle up with faith and take your compass of trust and start on your way. That blizzard will abate into just a few snowflakes, the sun will break through the clouds, and soon you'll enjoy moderating temperatures. You'll see beautiful landscapes, experience brilliant skies, and encounter new horizons. The journey will be worth it. *Are you ready to take the next step?*

*What are some of your fears about the journey of freedom? What unanswered questions do you have? Can you hold onto your faith and trust, and take the first step? You are not traveling alone. Your soul is always with you, and so are the souls of others who have gone before you. In the chapters ahead, you will learn the strategies of people who have refound the Freedom point, and the secrets of those who never lost their freedom in the first place.*

# the seven secrets of

# naturally thin people

Oh, those naturally thin people. You sigh with envy at the mere thought of them. You know the ones—they've never struggled with an eating disorder or weight problem, *ever*. They are at that healthy Freedom point with their bodies and their minds. No, I'm not talking about someone who is thin but is not taking care of her health, nor am I talking about someone who is thin but obsessive about her health. Remember the Freedom point. The naturally thin person I am referring to is at a weight that is right for her, a weight that regulates itself. And, while she doesn't worry about her weight, she doesn't ignore her body, either. You probably know some of these naturally thin people who have never struggled with weight problems, who live their lives in true freedom. You may look at them and think, "She's are so lucky," or, "I wish I had his metabolism," or, "Why can't that be me?" Why not you, indeed! *What would happen if you started to ACT AS IF you were a person who never had a weight problem?*

During my journey of freedom, I studied the habits of naturally thin men and women of all ages. I observed what they ate, when they ate, why they ate, and how much they ate. I took note of their exercise habits. I monitored how they spent their free time and how they lived their lives. I realized that people who have never had weight problems must have some secrets, and that if I learned these, perhaps I too wouldn't have a weight problem anymore. When I reviewed all I had learned, I discovered that naturally thin people really have only one secret—*they always listen to their intuition.* However, I noticed seven different ways in which they demonstrate this ability, which are the seven secrets provided in this chapter. *What would happen if you made these seven secrets your goals, learning to ACT AS IF you are a naturally thin person right now?*

## Secret #1: Practice Intuitive Weight Maintenance

*Naturally thin people have a stable weight and don't worry what it is.* If you ask a naturally thin person how much she weighs, she will say, "I don't know exactly, I don't weigh myself." She may get weighed at her doctor's office but even then it's just a number. Naturally thin people don't weigh, measure, or otherwise keep track of their bodies' dimensions. You won't even find a bathroom scale at the naturally thin person's house. If they are in the locker room at the gym, they walk right past the scale. They don't need to weigh themselves because they trust their bodies to regulate their weight on their own.

In contrast, when I was struggling with a weight problem, my life was one big, fat weight worry. And my weight was anything but stable. It fluctuated dramatically, ranging 55 pounds over a period of several years. I was on the classic weight roller coaster— up 10 pounds, down 5 pounds, up 15 pounds, down 10 pounds— and I wanted to get off! Those naturally thin people were not on this roller coaster, they were walking on steady ground. Sure, it was easy for them not to worry about their weight because their weight never changed. *Or, did their weight never change because they didn't worry about it?* What if my constant worries were *making* my weight fluctuate? What if my thoughts were so powerful that just the fear of weight gain made it happen? What if I tried to think like naturally thin people instead, *with an inner knowledge that my weight would stay stable?*

This seemed like a pretty good concept, until the fear set in: What if this is the weight at which I stabilize, or even worse, what if I stabilize at an even higher weight? Then I realized, even if that worst-case scenario came to be, at least I'd be off the roller coaster. No more ups and downs, which were so hard on my body. No more obsessing about how to get my weight down after it went up yet again. Just a constant, predictable, stable, healthy weight. Of course, I wanted my weight to stabilize at my thin ideal. However, I became absolutely willing to accept wherever my weight ended up. The most important thing was that my weight would be stable, and then, like naturally thin people, I wouldn't have to worry about it ever again.

In my work as a therapist, it doesn't seem to matter how thin my clients are; they all are usually worried about their weight. Interestingly, the thinner my clients are, the more worried they seem to be. One client, Jennifer, was pretty, intelligent, successful, and very thin. However, no matter how thin she was, it was never "thin enough." Her biggest fear was getting fat, which she had truly never been in her entire life. She weighed herself throughout the day, monitoring the most minute changes in her weight, and would often cancel plans to go out with friends if she felt she was "too fat." Finally, after I did some body image therapy with Jennifer, she began to experience her body differently, realizing she had been thin enough all along. She finally admitted, "I'm probably too thin," and became willing to trust her body to gain weight in an amount that was right for her.

In contrast, Andrea had been a dieter most of her life, and the more she dieted, the more weight she gained. With each size she lost while dieting, she would gain two when she went off the diet. She was feeling panicked at a size 24 (when she started working with me), terrified to trust her body, because her body was already obese. Andrea finally realized that her weight gain pattern was related to going on and off diets, but since she was no longer dieting perhaps she could trust her body. Andrea did not lose weight during the time I worked with her, but she *stopped gaining weight.* She noted, "A weight plateau is a major success for me, ending my pattern of escalating obesity. Of course, I wish my body would lose weight, and in time, perhaps it will. But if I stay exactly as I am, I'm OK with that, too." Some clients gain weight, like Jennifer. Others stay the same, like Andrea. And many others lose weight. Weight problems solve themselves when the weight worry is taken away.

*Can you trust your body to take you to the weight that is truly healthy for you, that you'll be able to maintain with no effort at all? What are your fears about letting your weight stabilize? What would it be like to ACT AS IF you never had a weight problem, and to let go of your weight worries completely?*

## SECRET #2: APPLY AN INTUITIVE ATTITUDE

*Naturally thin people have a positive view of themselves and their lives.* People who have never had a weight problem know that the key to happiness is in how they perceive themselves and their lives. They have a wonderful self-image because they have not allowed society's pressures to influence them. They can look in the mirror and feel great about how they look. Their attitude about themselves carries over to their whole view of life. They live from the inside out, letting a positive inner attitude create a positive outer life experience.

Sure, I thought, easy for them to do! They aren't overweight like me. Sure, I could be happy and positive all the time too, if I were just thin enough. In the midst of my resentment, it occurred to me that I had been thinner—and had not been happy. I wondered whether, even if I reached my goal weight, I would be happy. Then I'd have to focus on maintaining my weight, so I'd probably try to lose a few extra pounds to ensure a "safety zone." So, would I ever be thin enough? Would I ever be happy? *What if happiness needs to come before thinness?* I had been viewing it the other way around, putting the cart before the horse. But what if happiness was the *horse,* and the cart of thinness was in its way? What if I just focused on being happy, with no carts in the way, no strings attached, no contingencies?

I figured that naturally thin people could probably find something about themselves to rob them of happiness—maybe being *too* thin—but I observed that they don't try to dig up dirt on themselves. Meanwhile, I wasn't just digging up dirt, I was piling on manure. It was like I was carrying my own bag of manure around with me, smearing it on myself with every one of my negative thoughts or critical words. It was time to leave the shit behind—literally. It was time to carry only positive thoughts, like naturally thin people. If they could look past their potential flaws, then certainly I could learn to look past my perceived flaw of excess weight. If they could be happy right now—today—then I could be too.

In my work with my clients, I notice that there are many "weighty attitudes" that people carry around. Besides appearance, my clients criticize themselves for their thoughts, feelings, behaviors—*everything*. How they see their bodies is a reflection of how they tend to see their entire lives. It's almost as if they are looking through "dark-colored glasses," seeing everything in a gray, negative light. So I often work with my clients to examine some aspect of their lives without those dark perspectives, using this as a springboard to their letting go of body criticism. For example, Mark was dissatisfied with his job situation. He dreaded going to work in the morning, primarily because he believed he was not performing well enough. However, Mark's performance reviews were all extremely positive, indicating he was one of the best employees his company had ever had. I worked with Mark to reframe the way he saw his own performance, shifting from those dark-colored glasses to real 20–20 vision. With renewed confidence in his performance, he finally was able to enjoy his career and actually looked forward to going to work, which further enhanced his performance. Mark had also been extremely critical of his looks, but learned to apply the same process of removing the "dark-colored glasses" to see his self-image in an accurate, positive light. Interestingly, Mark's renewed confidence in his looks also carried over to his work performance. He noted, "I didn't realize how much my limiting views of myself were limiting me.

Free of my body worries, I am more focused, creative, and successful on the job and in all areas of my life."

*Have you been putting thinness before happiness? What kinds of criticism have you been carrying with you in your "bag of manure"? What positive thoughts can you carry with you instead? What would it be like to ACT AS IF you never had a weight problem and be happy, right now, today?*

## SECRET #3: KNOW INTUITIVELY WHY TO EAT

*Naturally thin people eat when they are hungry, but for other reasons as well.* They eat because their bodies need fuel, but they also eat sometimes even if they are *not* hungry. That's right, they eat sometimes even if they are *not* hungry. This was a major revelation for me. As a dieter, I often tried to eat only when I was hungry, but found this to be extremely difficult. Sometimes, eating for hunger only led me to go many hours without food because I could not detect my body's hunger cues. Also, sometimes I found myself wanting to eat at social functions even though I wasn't hungry, but I'd feel guilty if I did eat. I noticed that there are three reasons why people eat: physical need, physical desire, and emotional desire. Naturally thin people eat for all three of these reasons, with a proper proportion of the three.

## Reason #1: Physical Need

Physical need involves your body's need for fuel to function healthfully. Your body sends you various signs that it needs food. A growling stomach, an empty feeling in your stomach, lightheadedness, dizziness, or a headache can signal that your body needs to be fueled. The body not only sends signals that it needs food, it also sends signals about the *type* and *amount* of food it needs. If your body needs certain nutrients, your body will guide you to a specific food. If you have ever found yourself hungry and knowing exactly what you want, this is a physical need. For example: "I'm hungry. I could really go for a salad with lots of veggies!" When you eat out of physical need, your body guides you to the amount that is right for you. You will feel satisfied with your food choice. When you finish eating, you will not feel overstuffed.

## Reason #2: Physical Desire

Physical desire involves wanting to eat due to external triggers, such as seeing food, smelling food, or hearing others eating food. You may or may not be hungry when you eat out of physical desire. For example, you have already had dinner and you are watching television later in the evening. You see an ad for pizza, and suddenly find yourself wanting to order a pizza. Or you are on your way home from work. You have no idea what you want for dinner, but as you pass a number of fast-food restaurants, you decide to swing through for take-out.

Physical desire also leads you to make your food choices based on cost or convenience—eating what's on sale or what's most readily available. Another example of where physical desire can come into play is the buffet table. Rather than selecting what your body may really need, you will be swayed by how the food looks and smells as you peruse the buffet selections. Also, when you open your refrigerator or cupboard to see what's there to eat, and make your decision based on what you see, you are eating out of physical desire. It can be easy to overeat when you eat for physical desire, because the food appeals to the senses. "This tastes *soooooo* good!" you think, as you reach for more. However, it really takes only three bites to satisfy your sense of taste. If you find yourself wanting more, you may be hungry—or you may be reaching for food for an emotional reason.

## Reason #3: Emotional Desire

Emotional desire involves eating as a means of coping with your emotions. You may or may not be aware of the emotions that you are feeling. Any emotion can be a trigger, especially stress, boredom, frustration, anxiety, depression, guilt, fear, and anger. When you eat for emotional reasons, it can feel as if your stomach is a bottomless pit. It can be very easy to eat, and eat, *and eat* because there were never any hunger signals to begin with, and fullness signals are overridden. The comfort and security of eating is the only thing that matters at the moment.

As I thought about the reasons why I ate, I realized that on any given day I was eating about 75 percent of the time for emotional desire, 20 percent of the time for physical desire, and 5 percent of the time for physical need. My emotions were the primary reason that I was eating, and I was also triggered to eat just because the food was there. Very rarely was I in tune with my body's true hunger. So what was the answer? I found it impossible to eat 100 percent of the time for physical need, as suggested in many weight loss books. But clearly, the reasons I was eating were somehow out of proportion.

So, what is the proportion of the reasons why naturally thin people eat? I have observed that they eat 75 to 100 percent of the time because of physical need, 0 to 25 percent of the time because of physical desire, and 0 to 10 percent of the time because of emotional desire. This means that every now and then, a person without a weight problem will eat 100 percent of the time because she is hungry. But there may also be days when 75 percent of the time she ate because she was hungry, 20 percent of the time because something looked or smelled good, and 5 percent of the time because of stress. The key is proper proportion: to be attuned to the body's signals of what it needs, but also to eat once in a while out of desire. This involves using the body's *inner wisdom*.

Each of us is born with an inherent inner wisdom that guides us to the amount and type of food that is right for our bodies. Most children are in close touch with this type of intuition. Children tend to eat mostly because they are hungry. They never feel guilty when they eat, and they know to stop eating before they get full. This inner wisdom also guides our bodies to move in ways that feel good and enhance well-being. Children play for hours, running or riding bicycles or swimming just because it is fun and feels good. It is only when children learn about "good" and "bad" foods, about exercising as a way to burn calories, and about the pressure to meet society's "beauty" standards that they lose touch with this inner wisdom and develop various weight problems.

I spent years trying to "fix" my weight problem, only to discover that I needed to get back in touch with what I had left behind at age ten. I realized that the secret I was looking for was already inside myself. My body was perfectly able to take care of me, but I had lost touch with its message because of all the diets I had tried. What we need is already within us; to find it we need to reconnect with our intuition. Eating with inner wisdom involves eating mostly out of physical need, and making the food choices in type and amount that are right for us.

I suggest to my clients that when they find themselves thinking they'd like something to eat, they should "check in" first and ask *why* they want to eat. Is it physical need, physical desire, or emotional desire? Are there signs of hunger, or not? If not, what is the true "hunger" for—is there something besides food that would better satisfy them? If you realize that you have an emotional desire, then you may want to try to deal with your emotions in other ways. As discussed previously, it can be very easy to overeat when you feel stress, boredom, frustration, or any other emotion. Sometimes there's nothing like a big bowl of mashed potatoes or a chocolate chip cookie fresh from the oven to offer comfort during difficult emotional times. In *The Tao of Eating,* Dr. Linda Harper discusses the "soul of food," offering insights about why certain foods are appealing when we need to satisfy an emotional desire. Naturally thin people sometimes let themselves enjoy comfort foods, so give yourself permission as well. The key is to be *aware* of your choice. Make emotional desire a soulful experience instead of a guilt-ridden one.

The same is true for physical desire. Perhaps you're at a party, being tempted by all the wonderful foods on a buffet table. Seeing food, smelling food, seeing and hearing people eat food can all trigger a physical desire to eat. So if you know you are not hungry, but you just want to eat, scan the buffet table and select the foods that are most appealing to you. Sample a few different things, enjoying the taste of a few bites of each. Be aware, and let your food selections be a soulful choice. Remember, it is OK to eat just because you want to or because you feel like it. Just *be aware* of your desire, and ask yourself if you really must have the food you desire right NOW. I often find myself wanting chocolate, but I don't eat it every time I want it. I check in with myself to see if I really must have chocolate right NOW, or if I can wait until later. I remember playing the game of not eating anything when I went to parties. I also remember the feeling of deprivation I had leaving parties. It is so much more enjoyable now to be able to attend a function and sample the buffet selection if something really strikes my fancy!

The key is to make conscious choices. However, there are many physical desire traps—those instances when you may be hungry but you're using your senses rather than your intuition to make food choices, without even realizing it. For example, Larry always had the same breakfast every day: bacon, scrambled eggs, toast with butter, and orange juice. This is a classic example of a physical desire trap—repeatedly eating the same foods out of habit, because they are familiar or simply because they taste good. Gina got into another physical desire trap. She ate lunch every day in her company's cafeteria and picked not what she needed but whatever she thought looked good, smelled good, or would taste good. Alice, the president of her own corporation, often ate out and got caught in yet another physical desire trap. Because she was budget conscious, she'd scan the menu for the lowest-priced items and make her selection based on cost. Larry, Gina, and Alice were probably all hungry, but they were not responding to their *true* hunger. Each eventually learned to shift from physical desire to physical need by tuning in to what he or she was *really* hungry for, rather than eating out of habit, eating what looked good, or eating what was most affordable.

Like Larry, you may find yourself gravitating to the same foods time and again. Expand your nutritional horizons and try new foods. Experiment with new recipes, try new restaurants, buy foods that you haven't had in a while, and enjoy your "regular foods" prepared in new ways. You may discover a new fruit, vegetable, or other food that you didn't know you liked. You may also realize that you are bored with your regular foods and find new alternatives.

I found myself in the same pattern for lunch, day after day. Finally I realized that I was eating the same thing because it was convenient for me. I thought of other food possibilities that would also meet my need for convenience, and then checked in with my body to see which choice would be most appropriate at the time. If you are in a rut for breakfast, lunch, dinner, or snacks, and choose the same foods over and over, try to determine why. Is it convenience, cost, or tradition? Think of new ways to add variety to your food intake, to better respond to your physical need.

Remember, the key is proportion. Don't expect yourself to eat 100 percent of the time out of physical need. Naturally thin people eat 75 to 100 percent of the time out of physical need, and you can be in that range, too. It's fine to eat some of the time just because you want to, or occasionally because you're having a bad day. Enjoy that piece of cheesecake from the dessert tray, simply because it looks so good and you want to taste it. Have a custard-filled doughnut, because it's your favorite comfort food and you're feeling really stressed. Just *be aware* of what you are doing. Pay attention to why you are eating, and make your choices in a conscious, proportioned way.

*As you think about a typical day, what percentage of the time do you currently eat out of physical need, physical desire, and emotional desire? What physical desire traps are you aware of? What emotional desire triggers are you aware of? What do you need to do differently to change the proportion of the reasons why you eat? What would it be like to ACT AS IF you are already able to eat for the right reasons?*

## SECRET #4: KNOW INTUITIVELY WHAT TO EAT

*Naturally thin people eat exactly what they are hungry for.* They seem to have an inherent sense of what they really need, saying things like "I could really go for a chicken sandwich" or "My body is craving lots of veggies right now." They'll go out of their way to get what they are hungry for, even if it means making a shopping trip. If that's not feasible, then they substitute another similar food. When dining out, they seem to have a sense of what they will order even before they open the menu, and they often choose a restaurant based on the awareness of their true hunger. And, while eating, they are in tune with whether or not the food is satisfying their need, and they make adjustments in their intake accordingly.

In contrast, I always tried to eat what I thought I *should* eat, ignoring what I was really hungry for. Of course, what I should eat varied, depending on what diet rules I was trying to follow. Most often it was a "healthy" plan, in which I'd force salads upon myself and abstain from fat as much as possible. It didn't matter that I was so sick of salads I could barely choke them down. It didn't matter that I really wanted all those foods with fat in them instead. I ignored my body's messages, and tried to stay disciplined. Unfortunately, I'd feel so deprived from not getting the foods I really wanted that I'd often end up overeating all the "bad" foods that I had avoided. Trying to "eat healthy" was a losing battle for me.

Have you ever experienced this deprivation? You probably know the scene. You go out for lunch with a friend. You scan the menu to find the item that is lowest in fat and calories. During your scan, you notice the restaurant's special: lasagna, your favorite. You think to yourself, "Lasagna? Wow, that sounds good. Oh, and garlic bread comes with it. Yum! But, no, that has far too much fat." You find the heart-healthy section and make your decision. "I'll have the light chef salad," you say to the waiter, with a smug look on your face. You're feeling pretty good about your choice because it has fat-free meat and cheese, fat-free dressing, a fat-free roll—a total of only five grams of fat in the entire meal. Then your friend orders. "I'll have the lasagna with garlic bread," she says with a smile. You look at her and wonder how she can keep her figure and eat the way she does. Your meal comes, and the entire time you are gazing at your friend's plate as she eats. "Oh, this is wonderful!" she exclaims. "Do you want a taste?" "Oh no," you say, "I have plenty here." When she slips away to the restroom, you grab your fork and take several quick bites off her plate. "Much better than this salad," you think. You clean your plate, and still find yourself looking for more. You have a craving for something . . . but what? Meanwhile, your friend has left over half her meal on her plate. She takes it home with her in a take-out container. You are thinking, "I wish I had that to take home with me . . . that's what I really want." An hour later, you stop at a take-out Italian restaurant and order lasagna to go. You polish off the entire serving. Your craving is finally satisfied, but now you are overstuffed. Wouldn't it have been better if you had just ordered the lasagna in the first place?

As for the fat and calories in the meal, it all balances out. I observed that when naturally thin people ate "big meals" or foods that were "high in fat or calories," they naturally balanced them out by eating smaller portions or foods that were lower in fat for the rest of the day. It was as if their bodies had built-in food meters, registering when they'd had enough of one nutrient and needed more of another. Food is just protein, carbohydrate, fat, vitamins, minerals, and water. Our bodies need different amounts of these nutrients each day to maintain health; they use all the food that we eat to nourish us. Whether we eat a candy bar or an apple, our bodies will break the food item down into protein, carbohydrate, fat, vitamins, minerals, and water. Our bodies will then convert the nutrients into other substances to provide energy and to help keep us healthy. At a basic chemical level, our bodies do not care whether they get a carrot or carrot cake. Both will be broken down and used to help us function. Certainly a carrot has more vitamins and minerals than a piece of carrot cake, and the cake has more fat than the carrot, but over the course of an entire day these nutrient differences will balance out if we eat in response to our inner wisdom. If we eat the carrot, then later we may want something with more fat. If we eat the carrot cake, we may want something with less fat and more vitamins and minerals later in the day.

At first, it was hard for me to believe this. I figured that I'd always want the carrot cake—one of my favorites! Would I ever get enough? Not just a piece, the whole cake! Would I ever be guided to eat anything else? I was skeptical, but a story told by author Geneen Roth gave me hope. In her book *Breaking Free from Compulsive Eating,* she discussed the process through which she learned to eat what she was hungry for. Her body kept saying "cookie dough," so she ended up eating only cookie dough for several days in a row. Finally, after getting her fill of cookie dough, she found herself wanting other foods.

This inspired me to experiment with trusting my own inner wisdom. And so, the next time I was hungry, I asked myself what I was really hungry for. "Peanut Butter Crunch Blizzard," my body said. Was I sure? Was this an emotional desire? No, I was hungry. Was this a physical desire? No, nothing was triggering me to want this. I was really hungry for a Peanut Butter Crunch Blizzard. So off I went to Dairy Queen to get my Blizzard. Because Blizzards were one of my favorite binge foods, I set the boundary of allowing myself one Blizzard a day, if I really felt hungry for it. I'd order a medium size, and then I'd sit down and enjoy it. I finally reached the point at which I no longer wanted Blizzards as often. Once every few days. Once a week. Once a month. Now, it's about once a year!

As my clients learn how to eat for physical need, I have them "check in" with their inner wisdom. They monitor how hunger feels in their body, and they note how hungry they feel. Then they determine what they are truly hungry for. Sometimes it's just a sense of texture, temperature, or taste: "I'd like something crunchy and cold," or "I'm hungry for something creamy and sweet." Other times, it's a direct sense of the type of nutrients: "I really need the energy of complex carbohydrates," or "I sense the need for lasting fuel from fat."

With practice, my clients have become able to identify specific foods that will satisfy their true hunger. Betsy noted, "At first it was hard to tell what I needed because I was so programmed into what I should eat. But I just kept checking in. Sometimes I still don't know exactly what I'm hungry for, but I'm getting much more aware." Just as I craved Blizzards, many of my clients tend to gravitate toward their former binge foods or "forbidden foods." But over time, they find they start to prefer other food choices. Carol commented, "I couldn't believe it, but it really happened! My body actually wanted a *salad!* I've never *wanted* a salad, I always ate them because I thought I *should.* But now I'm really wanting nutritious foods!"

Try to determine the exact food that will satisfy your hunger. Check in with your body to determine what it needs. Resist the habit of opening the cupboard or refrigerator or freezer to "see what's there," because this will only result in your making a food choice based on physical desire, not physical need. Try to get a picture in your mind or an imaginary taste of the food you are hungry for. Once you know what you need to satisfy your hunger, then check your supplies to see if you have the ingredients on hand. If not, you can make a substitution that will be close in taste to what your body needs, or you can purchase the ingredients you need if a substitution will not do. The more closely you can satisfy your body's needs, the more satisfied you will be with your meal, reducing the tendency to overeat.

Your body will give you feedback about how the food you are eating is working for you. Pay attention to your mood changes, incidence of illnesses, sleep patterns, energy levels, and overall sense of well-being in response to the foods you are eating. Try new foods, and notice any changes. Switch from processed foods to whole foods, try more fruits and vegetables, enjoy more whole grains, and pay attention. Try more protein or less protein, more carbohydrate or less carbohydrate, more fat or less fat. Which works best for you? Does it depend on the day of the week? When you are under stress, do certain foods work better for you? When you are more active, is there a different combination of foods that works more effectively? We each have our own unique set of needs, and these can change from day to day. It is impossible to develop a specific formula that works for everybody every day. Discover what works for you, and find the variations you need to accommodate your unique lifestyle.

To further enhance the ability to respond to physical need, I teach my clients to monitor how their bodies feel in response to different foods. I ask questions like: How do you feel after eating a big hamburger with fries? What are your energy levels like? How long does this meal satisfy you? How does this compare to eating a chicken sandwich with potato salad? Or a gardenburger (a grain and vegetable patty) with a side salad? What about when you eat pasta with Alfredo sauce? How about with tomato sauce instead?

I tell my clients that it is important to try a variety of foods, so that they will be better able to make the choices that are right for them. I explain that any time new foods are introduced or omitted from their regular intake, it can take several days or several weeks to notice the full effect. One of my clients, Craig, tended to eat a high proportion of processed foods, with very few whole foods like fruits and vegetables. So he tried an experiment, introducing a variety of whole foods into his food intake. After a few weeks of incorporating these new food items, he noticed that his energy levels were improved, his digestion was enhanced, and his weight began to drop. He found that once he had willed himself to try these foods, he naturally started to want them in his regular meals. He commented, "I probably would have eaten bologna on white bread sandwiches forever. But now I realize that I feel better when I eat grilled chicken breast on a whole grain bun. And I learned that I like vegetables like carrots and broccoli, although I never used to eat them before. And I'm still experimenting with new foods, learning what really feels right for me."

*What happens when you make your food choices based on what you think you should eat? What are some of your "forbidden foods," and what would it be like to let this label go? How do you feel after eating your current food choices? What foods would you like to try adding to your intake? What would happen if you "checked in" with your inner wisdom the next time you feel hungry? What would it be like to ACT AS IF you never had a weight problem, eating exactly the food that you really need?*

## SECRET #5: KNOW INTUITIVELY HOW MUCH TO EAT

*Naturally thin people stop eating before they get too full.* They often leave food on their plates when dining out, because the typical restaurant portion is usually more than a body needs. When dining at home, they often finish what is on their plates if they served themselves, because they are in tune with how much food their bodies will need and only put that much on their plates. They don't worry about "portion control," because they know exactly how much food to serve themselves, without weighing or measuring anything, and without consulting nutrition labels to determine the appropriate amount to eat. A naturally thin person can even take a spoon and eat right out of a Ben & Jerry's ice cream container, then put the container away when they've had enough (yes, *without* eating the whole carton)!

At one time, I lived by portion control. There were various ways that I tracked portions: by weight, by volume, by exchanges. But the problem with portion control is that it does not account for the normal variations in caloric need that occur from day to day, so some days the portions were too big, some days too small, depending on how active I was. Eating based on portion control resulted in my getting out of touch with my body's inherent ability to eat the amount of food that is right for me.

In my physiology class, I learned that when one's stomach is empty, it is about the size of a fist. Typically, that was the amount of food I needed to feel satisfied. However, I also realized that some foods were more calorie dense than others, and I actually needed less of this type of food. For example, peanut butter is very calorie dense, meaning that it packs a large number of calories in a relatively small volume. In contrast, lettuce is not calorie dense because it has very few calories, even in a large volume. I also learned that it takes about twenty minutes for one's stomach to register signs of fullness. I realized that if I ate quickly I could easily overeat, especially if I was eating a calorie dense food. So I made a conscious effort to slow down my eating, until I began to learn how my body responded to different foods. However, now I can eat quickly or slowly; speed does not matter. I am aware of how much food my body needs, and I eat that amount.

I encourage my clients to eat slowly, paying attention to how they feel as they are getting full, and to learn how to recognize their fullness cues. Many clients say that it is helpful to minimize distractions (such as watching television) while they eat, so that they can enhance awareness of their body's response as they eat. One client, Janet, who is an avid reader, noticed that she tended to eat slowly while she read, but that she also ate more than she needed, often nibbling for hours. Eating while reading had become a pleasurable ritual for her, and she didn't know how to separate the two at first. But she tried eating her meal and then reading afterward, and found that this worked well, allowing her to tune in to her body more effectively while she ate. She noted, "I was amazed at how little food it took me to be satisfied. When I ate while I was reading, I consumed far more than my body needed, without even realizing it." Janet noticed that she missed having "something in her mouth" as she read, so she experimented with drinking hot tea and found that this satisfied her even more than food.

*How do you decide how much to eat? What else do you do while you eat, and how do these distractions affect the amount of food you consume? What would it be like to ACT AS IF you never had a weight problem, and trust your body's inner wisdom to help you choose the right amount?*

## SECRET #6: EXERCISE WITH INTUITION

*Naturally thin people enjoy a variety of fitness activities in reasonable amounts.* They exercise on a regular basis, without going overboard. There is consistency without compulsivity. They use exercise guidelines, but in a way that honors their bodies' needs. Some exercise for longer durations than others, and some work out at more advanced levels than others. Their bodies just seem to know how much exercise is right for them. But regardless of the level of conditioning, they all have some level of commitment to making fitness a part of their lives. Their bodies seem to want to move, not be sedentary. As for the type of exercise they choose, they focus on what they really enjoy. Some are runners, others bikers, others are into swimming or aerobics classes. They don't seem concerned about how many calories they are burning, they just want to exercise because it feels good. It seems as if they actually *like* to exercise—what a concept!

Exercise was anything but enjoyable for me. It was work. It was an obligation. It was a regimen. I really didn't like exercise; it was just something I knew I had to do if I wanted to lose weight. My motivation was the diet chatter echoing in my head: "Exercise, exercise, exercise! Burn those calories, burn that fat!" Just as I had memorized the calorie counts of various foods, I also knew how many calories were burned doing different types of exercise.

I never paid attention to whether I was enjoying myself; I cared only about how many calories I was burning. I'd think, "If I finish my sixty-minute bike ride, then I will have burned off what I ate for lunch, so I deserve to eat dinner." I'd count down the minutes until I could quit. And I'd always feel incredibly guilty if I missed a workout. There was a time when I exercised in some way every day. I dragged myself through my workouts. My body was telling me to rest, but I would not listen. There was also a time when I didn't exercise at all because I was getting no enjoyment from it. I rebelled against all my exercise plans and did nothing at all. However, my strength and flexibility were compromised, and simple tasks resulted in my getting out of breath. Clearly this wasn't the answer, either. My pattern with exercise is typical of people who are trying to lose weight: all or nothing.

Somewhere in between compulsive exercise and a sedentary lifestyle was *freedom*. My body was trying to guide me to that place of freedom; I just needed to listen. Watching the clock until I could stop exercising, enduring muscle fatigue, and feeling miserable while working out were all signs that I was doing too much. Loss of strength and flexibility, shortness of breath while doing simple daily tasks, and general apathy were all signs I wasn't doing enough. Not only was my body telling me how much exercise was enough, it was telling me what kind of exercise to do. I discovered that taking a walk in the woods, riding my bike, and other outdoor activities had more appeal for me than anything done indoors.

I am so thankful that I view exercise differently now. There are different types of activity, and each type does different things for our bodies. I began to look at activity from an entirely different perspective in terms of how it was helping my body. What did

I need to do to strengthen my heart and lungs? An aerobic activity, like running or hiking. What did I need to do to keep my muscles and bones strong and healthy, and to prevent osteoporosis? A strength-training activity, like light weight-lifting. What did I need to do to maintain flexibility and overall well-being? A flexibility activity, like yoga. The calories that were burned, I realized, were irrelevant. When I focused on being active because of the benefits to my body, I found that I was enjoying the activity for the first time. It just felt so good to be taking care of myself!

Your body wants to move; it was made to move. In the past, before automobiles and airplanes and microwaves and other conveniences, people were active in their everyday lives. Today, because we do not have to labor as intensely for our daily needs, we tend to be sedentary. Exercise has become a way to get fit and stay fit. One of the excuses that people give most frequently for not being active on a regular basis is that they do not have the time. However, if you choose to make fitness a priority, you do have the time.

Many of my clients tend to overdo physical activity, while others do not do enough. By listening to one's inner wisdom, the appropriate amount and type of exercise is revealed. With moderation as the key, I encourage my clients to *allocate the opportunity to be active* every day. They can pick the time of day—morning, afternoon or evening—depending on their schedule. The amount of time can range from twenty to ninety minutes, depending on their current level of fitness. Then, when the activity time arrives, I tell my clients to "check in" with their inner wisdom. What type of activity do their bodies need? Aerobic, strength training, flexibility—or rest?

Listening to the body's messages has proven extremely helpful for my clients at both extremes, compulsive and sedentary. To assist the process, I use an example from physics, Newton's Laws of Motion. To summarize: A body in motion will stay in motion, while a body at rest will stay at rest, unless acted upon by another force. In the case of a sedentary lifestyle, the opposite force is activity. In the case of a lifestyle of compulsive exercise, the opposite force is rest. In other words, people who are sedentary need to try moving more, while people who are compulsively active need to try slowing down or even resting completely.

One of my clients, Kathy, was extremely compulsive with her exercise, often working out for three or more hours a day. She was completely deaf to her body's message that she was overdoing it, until she attended a treatment center where all exercise was prohibited. Kathy elected to admit herself to this facility during her summer break from college, recognizing that she could benefit from the more intensive treatment of an in-patient setting. After just a short period of total rest, she was finally able to acknowledge how overworked her body was—so overworked that she was unable to even climb a flight of stairs. When she finally started to exercise again, she was sensitive to her body's messages, especially aware when she needed to slow down. She noted, "I'm exercising a lot less, and I was sure I'd gain a ton of weight as a result. But I really don't notice much of a change in my weight at all. I mostly just notice a change in how I feel. I feel so much healthier and balanced now."

Another client's activity consisted of, as he described it, "walking and lifting"—walking to and from the refrigerator and lifting the fork from his plate to his mouth. With the assistance of a personal trainer, Bob developed a beginner-level exercise program. He became fatigued and sore after very simple activities, which was a message that his body was underused and unfit. This motivated him to continue, and as his conditioning improved, his fatigue gave way to increased energy. He noticed many other benefits as a result of his increased fitness, messages to help him stay active. Bob said, "I actually look forward to going to the gym. Now, that's a first! It's not about *having* to work out, it's really *wanting* to." The key for both Kathy and Bob was to tune in to their intuition—it guided the way to an appropriate level of exercise, and this made the exercise *enjoyable*.

*What message is your body trying to tell you? Do you think you are doing too little exercise, or too much? What types of activities do you think you'd enjoy? What would it be like to ACT AS IF you never had a weight problem, and trust your body's inner wisdom to guide you to the type and amount of activity that your body truly needs?*

## SECRET #7: LIVE AN INTUITIVE LIFE

*Naturally thin people have truly fulfilling lives (and it's not because they are thin).* Thinness is part of their experience, but it is not the source of their fulfillment. They have meaningful relationships with others—friends, family, co-workers. They enjoy significant experiences in both their professional and personal lives. They focus far beyond the number on the bathroom scale, tapping into their deepest and truest passions—for example, careers and/or volunteer pursuits in which they are making a difference for others; leisure activities that offer opportunities for both challenge and relaxation; classes and other resources for intellectual, emotional, and spiritual growth. They truly seem to be living the "American Dream"—or are in the process of achieving it. But the focus is not on having material things, such as a big home or a fancy car. The focus seems to be on enjoying life, exactly as it is, and making the best of things, exactly as they are. With this attitude of gratitude, they seem to attract more good into their lives automatically, without having to chase after it.

Meanwhile, during all my years of trying to control my weight, I was caught up in what author Dr. Wayne Dyer has referred to as "the disease called MORE." More diets. More weight loss. More improvements in my looks. And, yes, more money, more clothes, more material possessions. If I just had *more*, then I'd be happy. And so it goes, an endless chase after the things of the world. It was quite eye-opening for me to observe that naturally thin people seemed to *attract* the things that I had to *chase* after. I felt like a dog chasing its tail, never able to catch it, running in an endless circle and exhausting myself in the process. Naturally thin people seemed to know that the tail was a part of them already, and that it would follow them wherever they went. They just moved in the direction of their desire, and the tail followed. They enjoyed the process of life, rather than striving to arrive.

As I continued to read books on personal and spiritual growth, I began to understand more about the attitude of success that naturally thin people seem to embrace. They possess the ability to move beyond society's standards of what life should be, instead following their intuition about what would offer true meaning. This is not about abandoning worldly things—giving up all possessions and goals—but rather, it is about giving up the *attachment* to worldly things. It means having a goal without being attached to the outcome of the goal. If the goal is achieved, great. If the goal is not achieved, this is still great. No attachment to the outcome. The focus shifts to enjoying the *process* of achieving goals, instead of only enjoying their outcome. In this way, well-being is not contingent on any circumstances. Well-being is enjoying life, here and now, in the moment. With this insight I realized that *in this moment, I have all I need to be perfectly happy.*

When my clients learn to enjoy the *process* of their journey of freedom, there is a huge shift in their life experience. I compare this to what happens when you realize that you've been trying to drive your car with the emergency brake on, and then you release the brake. All of a sudden you can move ahead, in freedom. Freedom is not the *destination,* it's the *process.* Freedom is not something to achieve, it's a way to be.

One of my clients, Laurie, was in the midst of some major life transitions. A single mother, she was considering getting remarried and was also looking into a career change. At first, it seemed as if she needed to "get her life in order" before her bulimia would be resolved. She was that dog, chasing its tail in circles. Her analytical mind analyzed and planned everything. But then she learned to listen to her soul rather than her head. She became more accepting of her situation and more present in her experience, amidst all the uncertainty. She achieved a sense of peace, even though many things in her life were still evolving. She discovered that she didn't have to wait to enjoy her freedom, she started living her freedom in each moment. As a result, her symptoms began to dissipate on their own. She became like the dog whose tail follows it wherever it goes.

*Have you been caught up in the "disease called MORE"? What goals or material possessions have you been pursuing? What would it be like to let go of your attachment to the outcome of these goals, and just enjoy the process? What would it be like to ACT AS IF you never had a weight problem, and enjoy the full, rich life you already have?*

—◦—

*Take a few minutes and reflect upon the seven secrets of naturally thin people. Imagine what their lives are like. Get a clear picture. Now, put yourself into that picture. See yourself living a typical day as a naturally thin person. Notice the food and exercise choices that you make, and how you feel as you enjoy them. Pay attention to the goals and activities you are pursuing, and how you feel as you are doing them. What is it like to ACT AS IF you never had a weight problem? Are you ready to live that life right now? If you can see it in your mind, and believe it can happen, you can achieve it. ACT AS IF what you want is already here, and then it will happen.*

# beyond the number

# on the bathroom scale

To ACT AS IF you have never had a weight problem implies living like a naturally thin person, in touch with your intuition. Your intuition is already within you. You don't have to learn it. You already know it. You just need to tap into it, access it, follow it, and trust it. To ACT AS IF means that you are *remembering what you already know*. However, you may need to *forget* the diet mentality first. This is the process of letting go of the "voices of the world" so that you can hear the "voice of your soul." The minute you think "I *should* lose some weight," or "I really *should* watch what I eat," or "I really *should* exercise more often," you cut yourself off from your intuition. Diets make us dumb. Diets put us out of touch with our intuition. Reconnecting is about eliminating what is blocking your intuition, all the "shoulds" of the diet mentality. Once you access your intuition and begin to live the process of Intuitive Self-Care, you've got it for life. No more constantly going on and off diets. You can just live in freedom forever.

Most diets involve a plan, a process of "doing." To practice Intuitive Self-Care involves "undoing." Imagine peeling away the layers of an onion to reach the core. Some of you may have more layers than others. But regardless of the rules, shoulds, and regimens you have layered around your core essence, that intuition is still there within you, waiting for you to uncover it. It's like when the sun is hidden on a cloudy day—it may seem as if the sun isn't there, but it's just that the clouds are blocking it. To enable you to enjoy the sunlight, the clouds must move out of the way. In her book *Eating in the Light of the Moon,* Dr. Anita Johnston emphasizes that recovery from disordered eating involves reclaiming our intuition. She tells a story about a queen who did not follow the advice of others and instead trusted her own inner guidance, thereby saving her kingdom.

We each can save our own kingdom—our *life*—by reclaiming our intuition. In reflecting upon my own journey of freedom and observing those of my clients, I discovered that there were seven strategies that we all implemented to dissipate the "clouds of our weighty attitudes" and bask in the "sunlight of our intuition." Incorporating these strategies into your own life can take you beyond the number on the bathroom scale to the Freedom point, where you can then begin to ACT AS IF you never had a weight problem.

Several years ago, following a workshop I had just given, a participant came up to me to tell me about her experience. She said, "I've been to so many diet doctors, and all they ever did was give me pills to take and meal plans to follow, which just made me obsess about my weight even more. But you're not like them— *you're the 'Don't Diet' Doctor.* As I listened to you, it was as if you were *surgically removing the diet mentality from my mind.* Now, for the first time in years, I can hear my intuition again." Just as a surgeon removes diseased areas from the body, I help remove "diseased" areas from the mind. However, I merely provide the process; it's up to each individual to become the "Don't Diet" doctor for him or herself, learning to remove the diet mentality. Many people expect that I will "fix" them, and I explain that they are not broken. I see my clients as already being whole—my job is to help them recognize that in themselves. You must learn to let go of what is blocking that awareness.

As a therapist, I guide others to find their own unique solutions. But not everyone likes this concept initially. My clients tend to want me to tell them the answers—what they should do and how they should live their lives—because it seems easier to follow my advice than to look for their own solutions. But I know that finding the solutions on one's own is the key to freedom, so when asked for advice I always say "Your answers are within." At first the answers can seem difficult to hear, but most clients begin to access their intuitive guidance within a few weeks. One of my anorexic clients, Mary, said, "I remember being so frustrated at first because I just wanted you to hand me the solution. But then I realized that the root of my problem was my impatience and my tendency to look to others—and diets—for how to live my life. The greatest gift I received was the one I gave myself, by going within for my own answers."

Once, during a media appearance, the host said, "So Dr. Dorie, what you're really saying is that weight problems are hearing problems?" And I said "Yes, they are!" But not hearing with our ears—it's "hearing" the voice of our intuition. Remember, a weight problem is not about weight. Weight loss does not determine success in solving a weight problem. A person may have lost weight on the outside but still be worried or obsessed about her weight on the inside. And in the case of anorexia, weight gain does not ensure success. Success means achieving one's natural body weight and balanced mental weight. Success implies freedom from the need to ever worry about weight again. Success is "losing your weight consciousness" and "gaining your spiritual consciousness"—the reconnection with your intuition. The seven strategies described here are the pathway to success. Keep in mind that the journey of freedom is not a destination, *it's a way to be.*

Some of my clients overcame serious eating disorders, while others solved chronic dieting or overweight issues. Regardless of their problems—from anorexia to obesity—these seven strategies were the common factors in their success. I have listed these strategies in the order that I applied them in my own experience. I don't believe the order is important—find the sequence that works for you and follow it.

At the end of each strategy discussion there are a few questions to ask yourself. In every case I ask, "What would happen if . . . ?" I commonly ask this question of my clients during therapy sessions. This question allows you to formulate a mental picture of the "if" situation. In this way, you can enter into the strategies to see how they feel for you. Imagining yourself living your goals is a first step toward making them your reality.

## STRATEGY #1: RELEASE YOUR FEARS OF FREEDOM

*People who are free are fully committed to freedom and all that it may bring.* At different points on my journey of freedom, there was a part of me that really wanted to be free . . . and another part that was *terrified.* It was like driving a car with the emergency brake on: I would move forward, but with great resistance. Sometimes the resistance was so significant that I couldn't move forward at all. Releasing the emergency brake—my fears—was essential for my success. One of my fears was that I might fail. What if I tried living like a naturally thin person, but couldn't? What if I was destined to have an eating disorder forever? Maybe it would be better to just not try, because then I wouldn't have to admit to myself what a failure I really was. After all, many of the books I had read suggested that I'd struggle with weight forever, and the best I could hope for was to control my symptoms. Who was I to think that I could really be free?

Thankfully, my therapist had a different philosophy, that *complete recovery was possible for everyone,* a complete and total freedom from eating disorders and weight problems. She was living this freedom, and she became my role model. With her example, I held onto hope that I, too, would recover completely. I let go of my fear of failure, telling myself that if she could do it, so could I. It almost became a pleasurable challenge, to prove that those other theories were wrong. I often imagined what it would be like to really be free. No more calorie counts running through my head. No more food rules. No more grueling exercise regimens. No more binges, no more purges. No more deprivation, no more starvation. I didn't know how to get to that place of freedom, but I held onto the hope that it was possible for me.

During a keynote presentation, motivational speaker Les Brown told a story about our perceived limitations. He said that if fleas are put in a jar with the lid on, they will learn to jump just below the level of the lid. However, if you then remove the lid, the fleas will continue to jump to the level where the lid was, *as if the barrier were still there.* At first, I was like one of those fleas, and most of my clients were like them. We had been told by so many others that we would never get better: "Once an eating disorder, always an eating disorder." "Obesity is a disease." "You have to watch your weight the rest of your life." These barriers can all prevent freedom—*but there is no lid on the jar.* I say to my clients, just as my therapist said to me, "Complete recovery is possible. You can live completely free of eating disorders and weight problems."

Rebecca, one of my clients who binged on sweets every day, said, "I figured the best I could hope for was just to control my symptoms. I thought I'd have to learn how to abstain from all my binge foods. You were the first person who told me that there was another way, and that I could live as if I never had this problem. Then I read about other people who had completely stopped binge eating, and now I really believe I can, too. I have the confidence that someday I'll be able to eat one brownie, instead of the whole pan." By letting go of her fear, Rebecca removed her barrier to freedom. Similarly, you have to remove the barriers in your own mind. Let go of your fear of failure. It is essential to believe that your possibilities for freedom are limitless. If you believe that you can be free, then so it shall be.

But what about the fear of being free—*the fear of success?* Bill, who was obese, noted, "I've been overweight all my life; what if I don't like being thinner?" For Liz, being overweight was a scapegoat. She said, "If I fail at something, then I can blame it on my weight problem. If I don't get a promotion, if I get dumped in a relationship, it's because I'm too fat. But if I don't have the weight problem, then what's to blame if I fail . . . except *me?*" Mary noted, "Anorexia is my way to get attention. If I let it go, will people still pay attention to me?" Barbara, who had been sexually abused by her uncle, commented, "If I succeed and I actually lose weight, what about all the extra attention I'll get? Maybe men will come on to me and I don't want that." Sally said, "My eating disorder is my best friend. Why would I want to lose something that's never, ever left me, that's always been by my side?" But once these clients let their fears surface, they were able to begin resolving the issues behind their fears.

I definitely was afraid of success. I was afraid of who the "new me" would be. My weight problem was familiar, but freedom was unknown. As much as I disliked my eating disorder, I also felt some safety and comfort in having it. For the longest time, my identity was weight, food, or exercise. I was what I weighed. I was what I ate. I was what I burned off. I was anorexic, a chronic dieter, bulimic, a binge eater, an emotional eater, overweight, obese. I used all of these labels to describe myself. And yet none of these was my real identity. But behind the masks of my "disease," behind the masks of meeting society's standards, behind the masks of who I thought I should be to please others . . . *who was I?* What if I didn't like my real identity? What if it required making changes I didn't want to make? What if it meant giving up a way of life I had always known? What if my real identity turned out to be even worse than what I had been living?

Or, what if my real identity turned out to be *better than anything I could ever imagine?* It's often said that our biggest fear is of *our own greatness.* It can seem easier to be mediocre than to claim our true essence. It seemed easier for me to keep that emergency brake on and keep my eating disorder, because I was so afraid of who I might become and the responsibilities of that new life. However, the conflict of not being who I really was eventually caused so much pain that I became willing to let go of my fear of change. I released the emergency brake. And then I heard gentle wisdom from my soul: "You are exactly who you need to be in this moment." I felt a sense of peace, knowing that I didn't have to rush the process. I could uncover my identity at a pace that felt safe to me, allowing myself to change and adapt without overwhelming myself.

Taking off the masks that cover up your real identity can be a scary process. It may seem easier to *not* know who you are, because then you won't have to change. Once my clients realize that change will actually help them feel better, they become willing to honor their inner guidance to let the changes unfold. Knowing that others have successfully made changes in their lives may give you some encouragement, so here are a few examples of the changes my clients made.

Hilary realized she was not happy in her relationship with her boyfriend, and she ended the relationship, took time to learn what a meaningful relationship would mean to her, and began the process of dating again. Lisa, a mother of four who was feeling a desire to be "more than just a mom," hired a part-time babysitter so she could have time to get a massage, have tea with friends, do volunteer work or other activities outside her role as a mother. Joan, another mother with three children at home, realized that she wanted to spend more time with her family, so she cut back on her hours as a volunteer. Mary, one of my anorexic clients who was mentioned earlier in this chapter, realized that a major trigger of her restrictive patterns was on-the-job stress. She ended up quitting her job and returning to school to pursue a new career that would offer her more work satisfaction.

Kathy, one of my bulimic clients mentioned earlier in conjunction with her compulsive exercise patterns, made a decision to let go of yet another rigid pattern—the pursuit of her college degree in "record time." She had planned to finish college in less than four years, but as her graduation date was getting closer, she realized that she was unhappy with her chosen major. Kathy decided to postpone her graduation so that she could take additional classes and learn about other fields of interest. As a result, she ended up changing majors to something that offered her more fulfillment, giving herself permission to graduate later than originally planned.

However, the process of making such choices can be difficult, because we often seem to have *too many* options. The fear that we might make the wrong decision can prevent us from making any choices at all. As Kathy was in the midst of choosing her major, she was overwhelmed by all the possibilities. She had a sense of what she really felt drawn toward but was afraid of what others would think. She was terrified she might make the wrong choice, which paralyzed her.

To help her through the situation, I shared an analogy with her. Imagine you are standing in a huge shoe store, with thousands of styles to choose from. You narrow your options down to a few different selections, and you try them on to see how they fit. Others around you say "Oh, I like that pair on you," or "You really shouldn't get those," which sways you in various directions. But ultimately you're the one who has to wear the shoes, so you decide to focus on the pair that really feels right for you. When you find that pair, you take it out into the world and see how it suits you. If it doesn't fit well after all, you can always go back and pick out a new pair. If you learn that new styles have just arrived and you want to see if you might like those even better, you can go try them on for size. There is never a wrong choice because you can always choose again. By applying this analogy to her situation,

Kathy was able to make the career choice that felt right for her, knowing that she could always choose differently later if she wanted to.

*What are your fears of failure? What "lids" have you been placing over your own healing process? What would happen if you let go of any limiting attitudes and beliefs about eating disorders and weight problems? What are your fears of success? What would happen if you allowed yourself to "try on some new shoes" and become who you really are?*

## STRATEGY #2: GET RID OF YOUR FOCUS ON THE PROBLEM

*People who are free focus on what they really want.* At first, I wanted to get rid of my excess weight. Next, I wanted to get rid of my eating disorder. Finally I realized that I needed to get rid of my focus on the *problem* and start focusing on the *solution*. I ask my clients in their first session, "What do you want as a result of our work together?" And they'll respond "To lose weight," or "To stop being bulimic." I'll reply, "No, that's what you *don't* want. What *do* you want?" Then they look at me, very puzzled, as I continue: "Weight is what you don't want. An eating disorder is what you don't want. So, what *do* you want?" As we talk a little more, clients begin to say things like, "Well, I guess I want to be thin." I'll respond, "OK, so let's say I wave a magic wand and suddenly you're thin. But you still feel fat. And you're still worried about your weight. So, is thinness what you really want, or are there some inner qualities that you're after?" Then they get it. They'll say things like, "I want to look in the mirror and feel good about the image I see," "I want to climb a flight of stairs without getting out of breath," "I want to have a completely normal and healthy relationship with food."

As my clients learn to focus on what they really want, I guide them to phrase their goals in a way that captures the *essence* of what they desire. Clients often become too specific with their goals, which can compromise their ability to achieve what they really want. For example, Linda realized that her primary goal was to be healthy. However, she was convinced that she would be healthy only at a specific weight. Her goal was, "I want to be healthy and weigh 125 pounds." I asked her, "What if you'll actually be healthy at 135 pounds, but 125 pounds would be too thin and therefore unhealthy for you? Or, what if you'll be healthy at 120 pounds, even less weight then what you thought you'd like to weigh?" Linda realized that being healthy was truly the most important thing to her, and that she would be limiting the expression of health if she stayed attached to her weight goal of 125 pounds. She decided to focus on health, and let her body's weight respond accordingly. Her goal became simply, "I want to be healthy."

Next, I have my clients rephrase their desires in a new way, using the word "choose" instead of "want." I explain that asking "What do I want?" can be a good way to tap into one's deepest and truest desires. However, phrasing the desire as a want keeps it suspended in the future, thus setting you up to always be wanting, but never attaining what it is that you want. In contrast, articulating the desire as a choice activates the desire in the present. It becomes your intention, not merely a wish. Using the examples from above, the rephrased versions are, "I choose to look in the mirror and feel good about the image I see," "I choose to climb a flight of stairs without getting out of breath," "I choose to have a completely normal and healthy relationship with food."

Over the years, I have noticed some common themes in the goals that my clients choose for themselves. The five most common benefits these clients have found or are working toward are: *happiness, health, balance, peace, and confidence.*

*What do you really want? What would happen if you chose happiness, health, balance, peace, and confidence for yourself?*

## STRATEGY #3: THROW AWAY YOUR SCALE

*People who are free feel good about their bodies and in their bodies.* I was at war with my body. I hated practically everything about it. I wanted to cut off pieces of my body because they disgusted me so much. I would punch myself because I felt so fat and I hated the fat. I could not stand to look at myself in the mirror. If I caught a glimpse of myself, it would send me into a downward spiral of negative thinking and self-criticism. A turning point for me was an experience I had while walking down the street one day. I happened to catch a glimpse of myself in a storefront window. The vision I saw was of a huge, misshapen person with oversized hips and thighs. "Ugh!" I thought, "I am disgusting!" The negative self-talk continued, and I became focused on my "cellulite-laden thunder thighs." Thoughts like "I'll never beat this" and "I'm just going to be fat forever" swirled in my mind. The more I thought in this way, the worse I felt. I couldn't even look people in the face as I passed them on the sidewalk. Feeling totally hopeless, I planned to stop off at the candy store down the street to get a big bag of chocolate to drown my feelings in food.

Staring at the ground as I shuffled along in my depressed state, I found my downward spiral interrupted as a voice ahead of me said a loud "Hello!" I looked up to see a man with a big smile on his face.

He was in a wheelchair, and I noticed that he had no legs. "Have a great day!" he continued as he passed me. I stopped dead in my tracks. A wave of emotion came over me, as if I had been plodding along in the desert and was suddenly engulfed by a large flood. Suddenly, the size of my "thunder thighs" no longer mattered. How my legs looked was not important. I looked up to the sky and said, "Thank you, God; I have legs." I walked past the candy store and continued home. As I walked, I noticed how it felt to move my legs. I paid attention to my unique stride. I was able to affirm for the first time many positives that my legs gave me. My eyes teared up as a flood of emotions washed through me. I felt incredible sadness as I thought of the years I had spent putting myself down, minimizing the gifts that I did have, unable to appreciate my inherent value. I also felt great relief, because I was finally able to feel good about my body. Then, I froze. Suddenly I realized that I was feeling good about my body, *yet I hadn't lost a pound.*

I realized that at every moment, I have two choices. One is to belittle and berate myself because I am less-than-perfect on the outside, according to society's standards. The second choice is to feel good about myself and accept the body I have at that moment, because at least it works pretty well. I realized that I had been putting my life on hold, and preventing myself from having the happiness I wanted. By learning how to feel good about myself in the present moment, I opened the door to happiness. I realized that I need to feel good about all the parts of my body: my arms, my legs, my stomach, my face—every part. A body image workshop helped me learn to appreciate the gifts that I have in my body, regardless of its size.

With my clients I find that body image therapy is essential. The first part of body image work involves feeling good *about* one's body, and the second part involves feeling good *in* one's body. The two parts actually go hand-in-hand; you can't have one without the other. Visualizations and art therapy techniques help improve body perception, while kinesthetic techniques help improve body sense. Many of my clients initially resist this body image therapy due to a common fear: "If I accept my body, then I'll stay fat forever." However, an interesting thing occurs with improved body image. *When you feel good* about *your body and feel good* in *your body, you naturally take good care of your body.* Clients who were overeating began to eat less. Clients who were starving themselves began to eat more. Clients who were sedentary began to move their bodies more often. Clients who were overexercising began to rest more.

One of my anorexic clients, Mary, who I have mentioned previously, was a prisoner of her own negative body image. She said, "With all of my self-loathing, I locked myself inside a dark prison cell. I thought the key to freedom was to get thin enough. I put my life on hold, passing up on so many opportunities because I felt too fat. I kept searching for that key, trying to lose weight as a way to be happy. But now I'm anorexic, and I hate my bony legs. I've discovered that thinness is not the key after all. I was too fat and miserable, and now I'm too thin and miserable. I'm still in a prison cell. But I have the key to freedom, and I've had it all along. The key is to accept myself in any given moment, exactly as I am. That means accepting my body right now, bony knees and all. With that awareness, instantly the bars of my prison cell have vanished, and I am finally free." From this point, Mary went on to overcome her anorexia, and she is now at a weight that is healthy for her. Accepting your body is the key to your freedom. This will open you up to the guidance of what your body really needs in order to be its best, and your weight will adjust accordingly.

Acceptance means releasing all body distortions. Anorexic clients tend to see themselves as fat, even though they are far too thin. Mary achieved her breakthrough because she was able to look in the mirror and see herself in reality as being too thin. Once she accepted her thinness, she was able to hear the messages of her starving body, which helped her to intuitively feed herself more.

At the other extreme, sometimes body distortions can occur with obesity. I have worked with several clients who were extremely fat and yet saw themselves as being thin. They were surprised when they finally realized their true body size, which motivated them to take better care of themselves. Accepting their overweight condition, they were more in tune with their tendency to overeat, allowing them to intuitively cut back on their food intake.

After having my breakthrough about appreciating my body exactly the way it is, I felt a huge weight being lifted away from me. Letting go of the self-criticism of my body lightened my load considerably. However, I had not yet let go of my ideal weight goal. I was accepting of my body, and yet I still wanted to lose weight. Every time I opened a fashion magazine or turned on my television set I was faced with yet another beautiful body, and a reminder of my own ideal—and how short of it I fell. Every time I walked into the bathroom I was faced with yet another opportunity to step on the scale, to check my progress toward that ideal. But no matter what I weighed I never had a good day. If the number on the scale went up I felt I had "completely failed," if the number stayed the same I believed I "didn't work hard enough," and even if the number went down I still struggled, thinking I "should have worked even harder" to lose more.

The same was true of recording my body's dimensions with a tape measure; no matter what the measurements were I was unsatisfied. Weighing and measuring my body was undoing all the good I had done to make peace with it. I realized that I was starting the war all over again. I had to stop weighing to keep the peace. My therapist had told me for months that I needed to throw away my scale; I finally understood why. Then my therapist helped me with the *how*. Since I had been weighing myself multiple times a day, I found it difficult to go "cold turkey" and stop completely. So I implemented a plan to slowly wean myself off of the scale, by cutting down the number of weigh-ins. When I finally stopped weighing myself altogether, I put my scale out of sight (and thus out of mind). Eventually I threw my scale out; what a release that was!

Clients who come to me with either anorexia or overweight problems are always surprised to see that I don't have a scale in my office. They are used to having weight used as a measure of their progress, and feel relief that they no longer have to go through the humiliation of weekly weigh-ins. But then they wonder, "How will my progress be measured, if not by body weight?" As much as they dislike weigh-ins, I find that many clients do want to check their weight as they go along. Overweight clients want to be sure they are losing weight, and anorexic clients want to be sure they are not gaining too much weight. But a watched pot never boils. *And a watched scale never changes. At least, not the way you'll want it to.* It can be difficult to let go of the scale and to trust the process as it unfolds, but this step is essential. As long as you keep weighing, you are hampering your progress. To quote an eating disorders Website, www.somethingfishy.org, "Scales are for fish!"

I encourage my clients to let go of the scale in a way that feels right for them. Some choose to gradually decrease their weigh-ins, as I did. Others stop cold turkey. Some bring their scales to my office for a scale-smashing ritual (an even better release than just throwing it away). After smashing her scale, my client Meg said, "My life was a function of the number on the scale. I was literally weighing my self-esteem. But now I'm free to be more than a number on the scale. This is the best thing I've done for myself and my healing—smashing my scale to smithereens!"

You may be wondering, if you throw away your scale, how can you measure your progress? The real changes that you are working toward cannot be measured with a tool like a scale, which only gives a record of a physical property of the body. Be aware that there are many substitutes for the scale—tape measures, fat calipers, even trying on clothes. Resist the temptation to monitor your progress in these ways. The changes you really want are occurring *within you,* and thus you can develop some internal methods of evaluating these changes. How can you measure happiness, health, balance, peace, and confidence? I encourage my clients to pay more attention to their moods, energy levels, and thought patterns. My clients often monitor their progress through journal entries, which show the shift from the diet mentality to freedom, reflecting emotions that are more clear and manageable and thoughts that are more positive.

*How do you feel* about *your body? How do you feel* in *your body? What would happen if you accepted your body exactly as it is right now? How often do you weigh yourself or record your body's dimensions? How do you feel after your weigh-ins? Does this help or hinder your progress? What would happen if you stopped weighing yourself? Are you ready to smash your scale?*

# STRATEGY #4: FORGET YOUR DIET RULES

*People who are free have made peace with food.* I was consumed with "diet mentality" thinking. I had calorie-counter books memorized. I knew the fat grams in most foods. If I ate "good" foods, I felt pretty good about myself. If I ate "bad" foods, I went into a downward spiral of guilt, frustration, feelings of failure, more guilt, and then a desire to eat in response to all these feelings. To remedy the situation, I tried to stick to my "good" foods. But my list was so restrictive that it was impossible to follow; I had far too many rules, controlled by my "goods," "bads," "shoulds," "musts," "oughts," and "don'ts." I was referred to a dietician for assistance in letting go of my eating-disordered attitudes, but her advice actually fed into my problem. She gave me an "exchange plan" to follow, which dictated that I select a specified number of servings of food from different food groups. This became just another thing to count, manipulate, and control. If she said I should eat six breads, I cut it down to three. This meal plan strategy did not work for me because it became yet another "diet rule."

Things finally changed for me when I took a nutrition class as part of my graduate school training. I learned the role that food plays in keeping my body healthy and functioning at its best. I learned about the functions of different nutrients: protein, carbohydrates, fat, vitamins, minerals, and water. Our bodies need a balance of all these nutrients. I learned how restrictive I was being to my body by following the various diets I had tried, and that I was disrupting my body's desire for balance by depriving myself of certain foods. I finally realized that *food is just food, there are no "good" foods or "bad" foods.* For the first time in more than fifteen years, I gave myself permission to enjoy *all* foods.

I find that my clients often have *too much* nutrition information, and this blocks their ability to practice intuitive eating. They *think* they know about nutrition, but their so-called knowledge is riddled with myths, misconceptions, and manipulations, just as mine was. I have noticed that my clients either obsess over nutrition guidelines or feel they are impossible to meet and thus rebel against them. For this reason, there are no specific nutrition guidelines provided in this book. If I determine that my clients do need more information about nutrition, I refer them to a registered or licensed dietician for education about the functions of various nutrients in the body. The key to nutrition guidelines is to use them *in parallel with intuition,* thus developing the freedom to enjoy all foods.

I work with my clients to challenge the nutrition guidelines that they have taken to an obsessive extreme. For example, many of my clients learn about guidelines for fat intake and assume "less is better," and many of them try to eat entirely "fat-free." One client, Sandy, who tried the "fat-free" approach, noticed that at first she lost weight. She talked with pride about the fact that she no longer liked the taste of fat. She was excited that she had "reprogrammed" herself to eat a low-fat diet. However, she reached a plateau with her weight, and she also noted that she always thought about foods rich in fat, even though she said she no longer liked their taste. Specifically, Sandy said she dreamed about eating cream puffs or butter-cream frosting.

Sandy's story is consistent with research on starvation. When calorie intake is cut dramatically, people have been found to literally obsess about food, especially high-fat foods. They will dream about food, and will often cut out recipes and photos of food from magazines. Because Sandy was not consuming enough fat, she began to obsess about foods with fat, much as people suffering from starvation do. She noted feeling hungry all the time, and mentioned that she snacked often (but always on fat-free foods). Fat in the diet serves a role in satiety, the sense of being full and satisfied.

It was not surprising to me that Sandy always felt hungry, since she was not getting enough fat. Her weight-loss plateau occurred most likely because she was consuming more calories than her body needed. It's a common myth that fat-free eating is calorie-free, but low-fat or fat-free foods do in fact contain calories. Sweeteners are often added in place of fat, so low-fat foods can contain more calories than the "regular" version of the products. When Sandy began to respond to her body's needs and started to slowly add more fat to her intake, she noticed that her obsessive thoughts of cream puffs diminished and her desire to snack also decreased. As her intake came to better match her true needs, her weight loss resumed.

As a client lets go of his or her diet rules, I find that "boundaries" are helpful. For example, Julie, a chronic dieter, realized she had become too restrictive about her fat intake, but she could not just immediately start eating higher-fat foods like French fries or cheese. She started slowly by adding low-fat products to meals, such as salad dressings or spreads. After adjusting to some low-fat foods, she then was able to add more variety, until she eventually claimed the victory of eating "real cheese"! Julie noted, "I was terrified of a piece of cheese. Terrified I'd instantly be fat if I ate it. But nothing bad happened. I really didn't notice anything at all. This gives me the confidence to keep trying other foods that I've been depriving myself of."

At the other extreme, one overweight client had a problem of binge-eating cookies. Rebecca, who I introduced earlier in conjunction with her bingeing tendencies, viewed cookies as "bad" and would never let herself eat them, which set her up to use cookies as a binge food. To break this pattern, she needed to learn how to eat cookies without overeating them. However, she was terrified to be alone with a box of cookies! I suggested that she set boundaries. She started out by going to a bakery to buy a single cookie when she really wanted one. She picked exactly the cookie she wanted the most and gave herself permission to enjoy it. As a next step, she tried buying two cookies, one to enjoy and one to take home for the future. When this worked, she tried taking two cookies home, then three or more, saving them for the future and eating only one at a time.

Eventually she felt confident enough to buy cookies in any quantity, and to eat more than one without it turning into a binge. Rebecca said, "I really don't even think about cookies any more. I know they're in my cupboard, but they no longer call out my name. Food has lost its power over me." Boundaries work until they don't work—in other words, if a boundary starts to feel too restrictive, it's time to expand it a little. Eventually my clients expand the boundaries so far that they can enjoy *all* foods, free of all their old "diet rules."

To make peace with "forbidden foods," my clients have learned that sometimes all that is necessary is to give themselves permission to have them. One of my clients, Diana, always viewed candy bars as a "forbidden food." Similar to Rebecca, she became able to establish a boundary, giving herself permission to buy a single candy bar at the grocery store check-out. She anticipated eating the candy bar, something she hadn't let herself do in years, thinking about how good it would taste. When she reached the car, she grabbed the candy bar to eat as she drove home. But before she opened it, she asked herself if she really was hungry for the candy bar *at that moment*. Diana realized that she could eat it if she really wanted it, but she decided to save it for another time. So she put it in her purse. Periodically over the next week, she would find the candy bar in her purse. She'd always ask herself if she wanted it at that moment, and the answer was still, "I could eat it, and it would taste good, but I don't really *want* it right now."

Another week passed, and she still hadn't eaten the candy bar. Finally, in the third week, Diana pulled the candy bar from her purse during her appointment with me. She beamed as she said, "I still haven't really wanted it. There were lots of times when I could have eaten it, but I realized I didn't even want it." Then Diana pitched it into the trash can in my office, stating she'd buy a new one if she ever wanted one. All she needed to do was give herself the permission to have her "forbidden food." She didn't have to eat it to be satisfied.

When you try to identify what you are really hungry for, do not let judgmental thoughts interfere. The thoughts might be that the food is "bad"—if so, remind yourself that food is just protein, carbohydrate, fat, vitamins, minerals, and water, and that your body needs each of those nutrients every day.

It is important, too, to remain *in the moment*. When I was making my food choices, I often found my thoughts drifting off to what I had already eaten that day, or to the plans I had for later in the day. For example, if I knew I was going out to eat later, I tended to purposely choose a lunch that was low in fat and calories. However, this meal was never satisfying to me, because I was making my present food choice based on either the past or the future. It is crucial to make food selections based on the present moment. When I found my thoughts drifting to the past or the future, I stopped myself and asked, "What am I truly hungry for, right now?" I tried to get a clear message, and to also picture the amount of this food that would satisfy my hunger. I often could see the food on my plate, in the exact portion that I thought would satisfy me. Then, with this picture in mind, I prepared my meal.

If you use nutrition labels to check for calories or fat, you will stay stuck in "good" and "bad" food attitudes. Make sure your food choices are based on your inner wisdom and what your body is truly hungry for rather than what the nutrition label says. You may have wanted that frozen dinner until you read the side of the package and saw that it had ten grams of fat! But ten grams of fat in the main entrée would be fine. Remember, your body needs fat to be healthy. Fat also plays a role in satiety, so without enough fat you will feel hungry all day. Rather than making judgments based on nutrition labels, pay attention to how your body feels when you eat specific foods and allow that feedback to guide you in determining whether or not you want to have that food in the future.

Perhaps you also consult the nutrition label to determine the serving size. However, what the box says is a serving size may be too much or too little to satisfy your needs. Rely on your own body to tell you how much you need rather than measuring or counting out a serving. If you glance at the nutrition label, look at the whole picture and get a feel for all the nutrients that are available in that food. Use nutrition labels to gain an appreciation for food as protein, carbohydrate, fat, vitamins, minerals, and water.

Dieters have been trained to count calories and fat grams. However, as long as you count, you will stay stuck in external measures instead of relying on your own body's inner wisdom. Develop trust in your body. Your body will guide you to foods with fat when it needs fat, and away from higher-fat foods when it has had enough.

To get my clients out of this habit of keeping a running tally of calories, I teach them a technique called "thought stopping." Whenever they start to count in their head, they are to immediately tell themselves "Stop!" as they picture a stop sign in their head. By interrupting the process of calorie- and fat-gram-counting, clients are able to unlearn a habit that had become second nature to them. Without all the numbers in their head, they are able to access their inner wisdom and to make food selections "in the moment," based on what their body really needs at that time.

*What are some of your "good" and "bad" foods? What would happen if you let go of those labels and viewed food as just food? What kinds of boundaries might help you to gradually step away from your tendencies to binge-eat or to restrict food, so that you can eventually let go of all of your "diet rules"?*

## STRATEGY #5: LET GO OF YOUR EMOTIONAL ATTACHMENTS TO FOOD

*People who are free express their emotions in healthy ways.* I had become completely out of touch with my emotions. It was as if I had built a dam to contain them completely; I had no clue what *any* of my feelings were. I didn't realize this was a problem until I was at a weekly support group session. One participant said, "I binged because I was trying to stuff down my anger." "Yeah, I can relate, " said another, "I was really angry too, and purging was my way to express it." I remember thinking, "Feelings? I *can't* relate.

My eating disorder isn't about *feelings*. Mine is about being *over-weight*. Once I get thin enough, then I won't have it any more." The discussion continued about how to express feelings in healthier ways, such as journaling, instead of using the symptoms. Feelings, feelings, feelings. Everyone was talking about the feelings that were behind their eating disorder symptoms. Then it hit me: I didn't have *any* feelings. None. I was completely numb. No sense of joy, no sense of anger, no sense of frustration. Just numb.

From this experience, it became clear to me that I needed to learn how to feel again. I was terrified of what this would involve, imagining the flood of emotions backed up behind that dam I had built. Therapy served as a safe environment for this process, as I learned to let the emotions come, a trickle at a time. At first, as my feelings surfaced, my symptoms became worse. I was a stress eater, a boredom eater, a frustration eater, an anxiety eater, an anger eater, a happiness eater . . . you name the emotion, I probably ate because of it. Food was a real source of comfort, security, and escape for me. When I ate, I felt soothed and taken care of. Although eating certainly did not solve my problems, it did keep me from having to face them. Unfortunately, the more I ate for emotional reasons, the more those emotions got stuffed away inside of me. I literally had to keep them stuffed down with more and more food. I didn't want to have to feel the feelings, and my symptoms served as a way to buffer what I was going through emotionally.

Then I began to understand what those people in the group meant. I could relate. I could see how I used binges to stuff down my feelings, or purges to try to release them. I could see how I used diets or starvation as a means to control something that felt out of control. All of the symptoms were my roundabout ways of coping. But coping didn't release the feelings; they were still inside me, waiting to be experienced and thus released. I learned that emotions would surface, but ultimately fade away. This gave me the confidence to feel my feelings instead of using my symptoms. The more I let myself feel, the less I needed my old symptoms. I learned to reach for what I really needed—a break from work, connection with a friend, a supportive message from a book—instead of food.

As I have guided clients through this process, I have noticed that their experiences are similar to mine. As feelings begin to surface, symptoms usually get worse. This can be terrifying, and can make it seem as if the process is backfiring. Overweight clients often eat more and gain weight, while anorexic clients often eat less and lose weight. But once they reach the point at which they really *feel* the feelings, not use the symptoms to stuff them back down, the symptoms dissipate. Overweight clients usually eat less and lose weight, while anorexic clients usually eat more and gain weight. Getting through this process can be frustrating, but the only way is *through*.

One of my clients, Cindy, had an emotional attachment to food, often gorging on potato chips and other snack foods during periods of stress. She said, "Food was my escape from reality. I used food to numb my feelings, but eventually this was more painful than the feelings themselves. I learned that my feelings really weren't so bad after all. Now I don't need food to stifle my emotions. I haven't binged in months."

At first, it can seem like eating is the most effective way to cope. Food can offer comfort, security, or an escape from the pain. However, food does not resolve the causes of emotions—it just hides them temporarily. I ask my clients to pay attention to their emotional eating patterns, to identify any situations that seem to trigger their eating. Then, we work to find alternatives to using food in an attempt to resolve those difficult situations. However, initially most of my clients are unaware of their triggers. They tend to work through this process in five steps:

- Step 1: Engaging in emotional eating, completely unaware of the emotional trigger.

- Step 2: Becoming aware of the emotional trigger, but only after having engaged in emotional eating.

- Step 3: Becoming aware of the emotional trigger, while engaging in emotional eating.

- Step 4: Becoming aware of the emotional trigger before engaging in emotional eating, but choosing to eat anyway.

- Step 5: Being aware of the emotional trigger and choosing an alternative to emotional eating as a means of resolution.

Dee Dee, one client who worked through this process, commented, "It's amazing. Stuffing myself with food used to be an automatic response to any intense emotions. Now, I don't turn to food when I'm emotional. I just use resources like writing in my journal or talking to a friend as a way to work through my feelings." Unlike emotional eaters who tend to binge on food, most anorexic clients cope with their emotions by *not* eating, while others will exercise for hours. The steps to resolutions are the same—just substitute "emotional eating" and replace it with "food restrictions and/or compulsive exercise" in the process outlined above.

Bruce realized that one of his triggers was the anxiety he felt about giving presentations at work. Before any kind of presentation, he had to exercise, even if it meant getting up at 3 A.M. to finish a workout. While exercise can be beneficial for some people to relieve their anxiety, Bruce was taking his exercise to an obsessive extreme. I suggested that Bruce begin trying relaxation techniques to appease his anxiety, in lieu of his exercise. He commented, "It still seems like exercise will work better, but I'll give it a shot. I'm tired of always working out so much." At first, Bruce preferred his exercise regimen, because it was familiar. With practice he discovered that relaxation worked more effectively, noting that he felt more alert and confident during his presentations than ever before.

Occasionally, emotions can be so intense that medication is used as an intervention. There are many antidepressants and anti-anxiety medications that can help resolve possible chemical imbalances. Psychiatrists and other kinds of medical doctors are involved in the assessment of whether medication is necessary, and they will prescribe the appropriate type and dose of medication. For more information about medication, consult your doctor.

*Have you built a "dam" to block your emotions? What roles do your eating, exercise, and weight symptoms serve in keeping your emotions "stuffed down"? What resources do you have to help you work through your emotions? What would happen if you let your feelings surface, and expressed them in healthy ways?*

## STRATEGY #6: DROP YOUR EXERCISE REGIMENS

*People who are free have fun with fitness.* Just as there are "diet rules" that can dictate what we should or should not eat, there are also "exercise rules" that can govern what type and how much exercise we should do. While the information that we have about fitness can be helpful in guiding us to make appropriate exercise choices, it can also be harmful if it is followed too rigidly. For example, I often made my exercise choices based upon what I thought would burn the most calories and fat. I developed a "more is better" attitude: If I read a fitness guideline that indicated twenty minutes of exercise was beneficial, I doubled it, and sometimes even tripled or quadrupled it. I outlined a rigid schedule, and if for some reason I didn't complete my planned workout, I'd double up the next day to compensate for what I had missed. I longed to have "runner's legs"—long, lean, and muscular. I pushed myself so hard to change my body and to burn cellulite off my thighs that I forgot how to have fun. I would look at my watch as I worked out, wondering "How much longer?" Now, instead of picking the exercise I think I *should* do for the duration I think I *should* do it, I ask myself, "What would I enjoy doing?" This allows me to actually have fun with fitness.

As with nutrition, I observe that most of my clients have *too much* fitness information, which interferes with their ability to be intuitive with exercise. One client, Holly, was compulsive about exercise, following a rigid regimen of aerobics classes every Monday, Wednesday, and Friday, with strength training every Tuesday, Thursday, and Saturday. On Sunday she usually did housework or yardwork. Her strict exercise routine was completely blocking her from honoring her intuition about her true fitness needs. Holly thought that unless she followed a rigid exercise schedule, she would not exercise at all. She explained that she had a busy work schedule, and insisted that she just could not be spontaneous with her fitness plans. I reminded her that the key is to *allocate the opportunity to be active,* and then choose the activity that the body needs at that moment. I explained that she could still schedule a consistent workout *time,* but that she could be spontaneous in responding to the *type* of activity her body needed.

To put this into practice, Holly continued to go to her gym on Mondays through Saturdays. When she arrived, she'd check the aerobics class schedule, walk around the room containing treadmills and other cardiovascular workout machines, and then glance into the weight room. She'd take time to "check in" with her body, to determine what type of available exercise felt the most appealing. After she had followed this scheduled-yet-spontaneous plan for a few weeks, we discussed how things were going. She noted that she chose to do aerobics about three days a week and to lift weights about twice a week, but that it felt better to have the flexibility of choosing which days to do which activities. After a couple of weeks, instead of going to the gym on Saturdays, she decided to try outdoor activities such as mountain biking. She commented, "It feels good to be spontaneous with my fitness plans. Now I'm attending new aerobics classes and am meeting new people, which is great. Plus, I've discovered a whole new world out on the mountain biking trails!"

At the other extreme, some clients find "exercise rules" too intimidating. They look at the guidelines of what they "should do," and feel that they'll never be able to follow through. Many of these clients have a history of failed exercise attempts, in which they would begin a fitness plan only to abandon it a few days or weeks later. They are convinced they will fail at any attempts to formulate an exercise plan, and so they rebel against exercise entirely. Other clients have grown up with negative messages about exercise, such as "Girls shouldn't sweat," or "Lifting weights will make you big and bulky." These clients have an actual aversion to exercise.

To change these attitudes, it is essential to look beyond "exercise rules" and just think about being *active* in very simple ways. I encourage these clients to use the word "activity" instead of "exercise," because activity implies simply moving the body. Clients realize it's pretty easy to do that. They learn to give themselves credit for day-to-day activities like climbing the stairs, standing up from a chair, or reaching to put a dish in the cupboard. Richard, who found aerobic exercise to be "too much work," discovered that he enjoyed gentle activities like yoga. Several weeks after starting a yoga class, he added walking as another activity. He said "I may never be a marathon runner, but I'm healthier than I've ever been! I'm so glad I realized I could do just a little bit at a time."

*What is your current exercise routine? What "exercise rules" have you been trying to follow—or avoid? If you've been compulsive, what would it be like to be more spontaneous? If you've been sedentary, what kinds of activities could you do to start slowly? What would happen if you moved beyond the rules, learning to do the type and amount of exercise you truly enjoy?*

## STRATEGY #7: ELIMINATE YOUR OTHER OBSTACLES

*People who are free surround themselves with supportive people and activities.* I tell my clients that the journey of freedom is like climbing a mountain. And on this journey, there are people climbing with you. Some are ahead of you, reaching their hand down to help you climb higher. Others are next to you, and you are helping each other to move to the next level. And then there are those who are behind you. Some give your foot a gentle tap, hoping you'll reach down and help them to climb up with you. But others will grab onto your ankle with a tight grip, and try to pull you back down with them. *These "ankle grabbers" do not want you to change and they will try to sabotage your best efforts.*

You have to realize which people in your life are which types of climbers. It can be hard to move away from those "ankle grabbers," but your success depends on it. You can love those people, but from a safe distance. Angela said, "But what if that ankle grabber is my husband?" She didn't want that safe distance to imply getting a divorce. She learned that she could create a safe distance by asking her husband not to comment about her weight or eating habits. And she placed extra emphasis on finding climbers who were at her level or slightly ahead of her, to whom she could turn for the support she needed.

In addition to setting healthy boundaries with people, it's important to be selective about activities. Our society is built around achievement. Those who do the most get praised. Hard work earns good grades in the academic world, promotions in the work world, and more possessions in the material world. Therefore, it can be easy to say "yes" to every activity that seems to offer the chance to achieve more. However, achieving more in the world can be a barrier to achieving freedom. I realized that the time and energy I was putting into my worldly pursuits was taking away from the energy I needed for my own journey of freedom. So I began setting boundaries and learning to say "no" to activities that I thought were "ankle grabbers," while still saying "yes" to those that I sensed would enhance my personal and spiritual growth.

Initially, my clients tend to struggle with this concept. Kathy, who has been discussed previously in conjunction with overcoming her bulimia, was afraid to say "no" to activities because she didn't want any unstructured time. Even if she felt exhausted by everything she was doing, this was better than being faced with free time, which she believed was "a waste of time." She couldn't imagine "just sitting there doing nothing." She had her days planned out to the minute, and she showed me the color-coded schedule that she lived by. Red was a school activity, blue a work activity, green an exercise activity, and so on. I had Kathy experiment with "scheduling unscheduled time" during which she could watch television, read, or engage in some other leisure activity. This way she could still feel she was *doing something* with her free time. Eventually she was able to schedule in more unscheduled time, and then finally she was able to abandon her schedule, trusting that she could enjoy free time as she needed it. Even though Kathy still felt compelled to *do something* during her free time, at least she was giving herself permission to have it.

Even when I wasn't *doing something* physically, I was *doing something* mentally. It seemed as if there was a constant stream of chatter in my mind. I was worrying about the future or rehashing the past, unable to enjoy *being* in the present moment. Eventually I found nature to be especially helpful in letting go of my constant mind chatter. It was hard to hold on to distractions when I was surrounded by nature and its beauty. I began to notice the trees, flowers, birds, and life all around me. The past and the future were not of immediate import. I was just enjoying the present. And in those moments of silence, I began to hear the voice of my soul speaking very clearly. By letting go of my diet mentality, and all my other distractions, I found my core essence. I have received some of my most incredible intuitive guidance while on nature hikes. I discovered that my hikes are actually a form of meditation. There are many different ways to practice meditation—all involve quieting the chatter of the mind, and sinking deeply into the stillness and quiet within oneself. *Be still and know the voice of your soul. Be still and know. Be still. Be.*

*Who are the supportive people and what are the supportive activities in your life? Who and what are the "ankle grabbers" that you need to create a safe distance from? How can you do this? What helps you to quiet the chatter in your mind? What would happen if you started to "do" less and "be" more?*

———

*Take a few minutes and reflect upon the seven strategies of people who are free. Which strategy do you feel intuitively guided to begin with? Are there some strategies that you are already implementing? What would happen if you applied all seven strategies in your life, at the pace that feels right for you?*

# living free of

# weight problems

It may seem that naturally thin people have it easy. After all, they are *already in touch* with their intuition, while you've got to *get* in touch with yours. You may be wondering if this is really possible, and what will happen as you try. What if it seems as if there isn't enough structure as you learn the process of Intuitive Self-Care? What if you still want to hold on to some of your old dieter's games? What if you can't seem to get in touch with your hunger or fullness levels? What if you try on your favorite pair of jeans and you notice they're getting *tighter?*

My clients have asked these same questions, and found the answers during the journey of freedom. I'd like to share four case studies with you, to illustrate what this journey is like. These case studies represent what I observe in my counseling practice to be the four archetypal weight problems. In Chapter 4, I defined weight problems as beginning in the mind with "mental weight" and then manifesting on the body as "body weight." As you will recall, "mental weight" can range from complacent/apathetic at one extreme to worried/obsessive at another, while "body weight" can range from underweight/anorexic to overweight/obese. The four archetypal weight problems reflect specific combinations of "mental weight" and "body weight."

The most common archetype that I observe in my clients is "Rigid Rachel," which reflects a worried/obsessive and underweight/anorexic combination. "Rigid Rachel" types are almost always worried about weight, eating, or exercise. Life revolves around reaching or maintaining an overly thin ideal body weight.

The next most common type in my clinical practice is "Searching Sarah," which reflects a worried/obsessive and overweight/obese combination. "Searching Sarah" types are the classic yo-yo dieters, who, having tried countless methods of weight control, have found none effective in keeping weight off. Overeating or binge eating often occur between their bouts of dieting, contributing to the yo-yo effect on their weight.

The third type is "Escapist Eric," which reflects a complacent/apathetic and overweight/obese combination. "Escapist Eric" types have often made the assumption that they will be "fat forever," and give little regard to nutrition and exercise. This tends to occur as a result of rebellion against years of dieting.

The fourth type is "Busy Beth," which reflects a complacent/apathetic and underweight/anorexic combination. "Busy Beth" types are often workaholics who do not take time for meals or adequate exercise. Although these types appear thin, they are usually highly stressed and suffer other health consequences.

Looking back, I realize that I have been all four archetypes at various points in my life. I started out as "Rigid Rachel," worried about weight when I really didn't need to, becoming anorexic and yet still thinking I needed to lose more weight. Then, in my late high school years as my weight increased, I was still frantically looking for the answer to my weight problems as "Searching Sarah." Finally sick and tired of all the weight loss games, I became Escapist Eric: I figured I might as well just give up and be "fat forever," not really caring what I ate or whether or not I exercised. I rotated among these three for more than fifteen years before beginning my journey of freedom. I started practicing the concepts of Intuitive Self-Care, and as a result, my weight decreased. But then I took my freedom for granted. I got busy in my work and with other pursuits. I became "Busy Beth," maintaining my weight but not necessarily eating the most nutritious foods, nor exercising in the amounts my body needed. Often I would open a can of Spaghetti-O's for lunch, eating right out of the can to minimize the disruption of my busy day. And, if I went for a workout, it was usually very short. I rationalized my behavior because I knew that my body's weight was stable. But then I had a standard blood test done during my annual checkup, and I discovered that my cholesterol levels were elevated. This helped me to realize that even though I was slim, I wasn't healthy.

I notice that many of my clients have, like me, demonstrated characteristics of more than one archetype. Over years of dieting and quitting, experiencing weight loss and weight gain, many of my clients have also resembled each of the four archetypes at different points in their lives. Most commonly, I observe that "Rigid Rachel" can become "Busy Beth," and "Searching Sarah" can become "Escapist Eric." The trend here is that when the obsessive tendencies of rigid weight control are abandoned or rebelled against, they are replaced with complacency. Be aware of your own tendency to shift from archetype to archetype. And, as you learn the process of Intuitive Self-Care and reach the Freedom point, be aware that you can slip back into any of the archetypes again if you take your freedom for granted. Intuitive Self-Care isn't something that you *do* until you reach a goal weight. It's a way to *be* for the rest of your life. This means making a commitment to your ongoing success.

## WHICH ARCHETYPE ARE YOU?

Review the checklist below to determine which of the four archetypal weight profiles you resemble most closely. As you make your assessment, consider the archetype's Body Size and Primary Attitude, as well as Food, Weight, and Body Worries. If you have characteristics of more than one archetype, you may be in the midst of changing from one archetype to another. Pick the one that seems to be the closest fit for you.

### Rigid Rachel

Body Size: Ranges from anorexic to average weight.

Primary Attitude: *There's got to be a way for me to lose this weight!*

Food, Weight, and Body Worries (possess five or more):

Counting calories, carbohydrate grams, etc.

Thinking about food nearly all the time.

Keeping a food diary, recording eating and exercise each day.

Avoiding certain foods (e.g., chocolate) or food groups (e.g., fat).

Restrictive eating patterns (small food portions, meal skipping).

Bingeing patterns (eating large amounts of food, often "forbidden foods").

Purging patterns (exercise, vomiting, laxatives, etc., to "get rid of" food).

Episodes of binge eating followed by purging or fasting.

Loading up on special vitamin/mineral supplements.

Taking appetite suppressants, metabolic boosters, etc.

Always "feeling fat," or being terrified of "getting fat."

Wanting to lose anywhere from 1 to 30 pounds.

Trying to maintain weight within a five pound range.

Checking body weight at least once a day.

Maintaining a record of body's measurements.

Being dissatisfied with body's shape and size.

Using exercise to burn calories or fat, or to change shape of body.

Exercising once or more every day, usually more than 90 minutes daily.

Feeling guilty if a workout is missed.

## Searching Sarah

Body Size: Ranges from average weight to obesity.

Primary Attitude: *There's got to be a way for me to lose this weight!*

Food, Weight, and Body Worries (possess five or more):

Having tried ten or more different methods to lose weight.

Eating is regulated by diets or meal plans suggested for weight loss.

Thinking about food nearly all the time.

Keeping a food diary, recording eating and exercise each day.

Bingeing patterns (eating large amounts of food, often "forbidden foods").

Purging patterns (exercise, vomiting, laxatives, etc., to "get rid of" food).

Episodes of binge eating followed by purging or fasting.

Having a tendency to overeat or binge, especially at emotional times.

Loading up on special vitamin/mineral supplements.

Taking appetite suppressants, metabolic boosters, etc.

Having lost and gained back 20 or more pounds.

Wanting to lose 20 or more pounds.

Checking body weight at least once a day.

Having had or considered liposuction or other weight-loss surgery.

Maintaining a record of body's measurements.

Being dissatisfied with body's shape and size.

Using exercise to burn calories or fat, or to change shape of body.

Exercising on a strict schedule, or not at all.

## Escapist Eric

Body Size: Ranges from average weight to obesity.

Primary Attitude: *Who cares about weight?*

Food, Weight, and Body Worries (possess five or more):

Past history of weight loss attempts.

Being resolved to "never diet again."

"Eating anything," ignoring nutritional content and weight gain.

Eating a high proportion of fast foods and processed foods.

Eating few fruits and vegetables or whole grain foods.

Nibbling on food throughout the day.

Having a tendency to overeat or binge, especially at emotional times.

Episodes of binge eating followed by "sleeping it off."

Having lost and gained back 20 or more pounds.

Weight loss not currently a priority.

Not caring about body weight or body's measurements.

Disliking exercise, seeing it as "too hard."

Having no consistent exercise plans.

## Busy Beth

Body Type: Ranges from anorexic to average weight.

Primary Attitude: *Who cares about weight?*

Food, Weight, and Body Worries (possess 5 or more):

Past history of eating disorders.

Food not a priority, often will "forget to eat."

Eating a high proportion of fast foods and processed foods.

Eating few fruits and vegetables or whole grain foods.

Having a tendency to skip meals, especially at emotional times.

Weight loss not currently a priority.

Not caring about body weight or body's measurements.

Having no consistent exercise plans.

*Which archetype most closely resembles you right now? Are there additional characteristics that you would add to any of the archetypes? Over the years, how has your archetype changed?*

## WHAT WILL YOUR JOURNEY OF FREEDOM BE LIKE?

The following case studies provide detailed profiles of four of my clients who fit an extreme example of each archetype. I have chosen to illustrate these extremes so that you can develop the confidence of realizing, "If she was in such a bad place and she can succeed, so can I." Each case study also includes three journal entries, which are composites taken from conversations with and letters I have received from clients at the beginning, middle, and conclusion of their work with me. As you read these journal entries, let your archetype's voice become your voice, and try to resolve any fears and doubts you may have. Walk with your archetype and discover what a typical journey of freedom is like. Some clients complete their work with me in as little as three months, while others take as long as three years, with an average duration of approximately one year. While some clients still yearn for a "quick fix," most recognize that it took a lifetime to develop their weight problems so they are willing to invest a year or more to be free. Be patient with yourself as you take your journey, and use your archetype's success as encouragement along the way.

### Rigid Rachel

When Rachel entered my office, I observed a very slender, well-dressed, attractive woman. She forced a smile as she greeted me, but this was almost immediately replaced by a pained look. Rachel was twenty-three years old, and at 5'5" and 109 pounds, she described feeling extremely overweight. She told me that she wanted to weigh 99 pounds, and she was willing to do almost anything to reach this goal. A waitress, she was around food nearly all day long, often working double shifts to earn extra money. However, she rarely ate at the restaurant where she worked, often fasting twelve hours or more each day, indicating that she got a sense of strength from serving meals to others while she skipped hers.

Rachel subsisted largely on diet cola, and said that she was taking a variety of herbal weight-loss products to help control her appetite. When she did eat, she preferred salads, steamed vegetables, and other dishes that she perceived to be low in calories and fat. Rachel said that about once a week she'd be so hungry that she would "eat everything in sight," but then would force herself to regurgitate afterward. Each morning she'd go running for an hour, then do hundreds of abdominal crunches. On evenings when Rachel had plans to go out with friends, she would fast all day in preparation, and if she still felt "too fat" she would cancel her plans. Rachel recalled starting her first diet at the age of twelve "because all her friends were doing it," and had been worried about her weight ever since.

### Initial-Session Journal Entry:

I feel like such a fat pig. If I could just lose another 10 pounds, then I'd be thin enough. Well, maybe 20, just to be on the safe side. Some people say that I'm already too thin, but I don't believe them. Liars. If I'm thin, why do I feel so fat? I've got to get rid of this weight! Whatever it takes! The problem is, I've tried everything

I can think of. I'm running out of ideas. And life's just not fun any more.

I'm constantly thinking about food. The calories are always running in my head. I don't even hear what people say sometimes because I'm too busy thinking about what I just ate, when I can exercise it off, and what I can eat next. I binge sometimes, and then purge to get rid of what I just ate. Some people tell me that I'm going to die by doing all of this. Sometimes I don't care if I die, as long as I'm thin in the coffin. I know this isn't normal. I know I need help. I just want to live a normal life again . . .

### Initial Steps on the Path:

Because Rachel had been trying to lose weight for more than eleven years, her "diet mentality" was firmly rooted and was blocking access to her intuitive voice. Her weight loss obsession was reflected in a collage she had made, covered with photos of her "ideal" body and words to inspire her weight loss efforts. She idolized this collage, and weight loss had become her worship. Her distorted body image was feeding her obsessive quest.

Our primary work involved body image therapy, in which Rachel learned to improve her view *about* her body and to experience a positive sense of being *in* her body. With an enhanced sense of body awareness, Rachel was then able to start tuning in to her hunger and fullness signals, while learning to challenge her old "diet rules." Concurrently, we explored Rachel's values, beliefs, dreams, and goals—beyond the number on the bathroom scale.

### Midway-Session Journal Entry:

What an eye-opening experience to realize that I'm really not fat after all. I had just convinced myself I was fat, and so I always felt fat. My body's not perfect, but it doesn't have to be. I can finally see the ideal standard that I've been trying to live up to. My poor body. I had no idea how much I was starving it with diets and punishing it with exercise. I am really trying to take better care of myself now.

It's been several weeks since I've binged or purged. Sometimes I eat more than my body needs, but I try to be forgiving. This is all good, I know, but my body has been gaining weight, and that is so scary! My favorite pair of pants doesn't fit any more. I had to go out and buy a few new things in a bigger size and I hate that! But, I am trying really hard to trust that my body knows the weight that's right for it. If it means buying a new wardrobe, then so be it. That's better than trying to cram myself into a size that is too small for me after all.

So, I'm trying to just stay focused on taking care of myself. I'm trying to deal with the issues that were underlying all of my focus on food and weight. And as I do, I notice that I'm starting to feel better about myself and my life . . .

### Midway Steps on the Path:

As Rachel gained some weight, her "diet mentality" was triggered. We continued to challenge each "diet rule" she was grappling with, and I also emphasized self-awareness. I encouraged Rachel to keep tuning in to her body's needs—what her soul (intuition) wanted for her body, instead of what her head wanted ("diet rule"). Each week, Rachel reported an enhanced intuitive sense about her eating and exercise. Rachel also continued to learn more about her true identity. She discussed plans to reduce her work as a waitress to part-time so that she could attend college and earn her degree in psychology.

**Concluding-Session Journal Entry:**

It's awesome, I am so happy! So much of my life has been wasted worrying about weight and how I look. Now I have found a better path. I went running this morning, not because I should, not because I will feel guilty if I miss it, but because I can and it makes me feel so good first thing in the morning. I have not forgotten to take a day of rest, nor am I overdoing it. I think that's what I hated before—I overdid it, then didn't want to keep working that hard all the time. I have emotionally eaten a few times, but I knew I was doing it. It feels like a soulful choice, and I honor that. I'm not completely free, but I'm very close. I feel like I can make it on my own now . . .

**Final Steps on the Path:**

During her final session, Rachel shared a new collage she had made. With a smile—a radiantly authentic one—she showed it to me. It was highlighted with pictures of children, a home, and other things that represented her dreams of the future. Rachel then identified strategies to reinforce what she had learned during our year of work together. I encouraged her to implement these strategies on a regular basis, and to stay aware of any "diet rules" that could return to thwart her progress. We discussed that the journey of freedom is a way of *being*, involving the practice of Intuitive Self-Care for the rest of one's life.

## Searching Sarah

Sarah started working with me after attending my workshop, "The Don't Diet Solution." She told me that she had come to the workshop by "total coincidence," and had planned to sign up for a new program at a local weight loss center later that afternoon. However, during the workshop, as she "weighed" the effects of all the weight loss games she had played over the years, Sarah realized that she wanted to stop dieting and start living again.

At 5'5" and more than 200 pounds, Sarah fit the profile of "diet-induced obesity," noting that each time she lost weight she regained it all, plus several extra pounds. She was uncertain of her exact weight noting that she was afraid to know "how fat she really was."

Sarah was a thirty-eight-year-old mother of three, who also had a career as a nurse. She expressed frustration about having been trained in a health field, yet not knowing how to manage her own weight problem. Sarah said that she had never tried to lose weight until after the birth of her first child ten years earlier. Since that time, she had tried "everything under the sun" to reach her goal weight of 125 pounds. She had reached this goal twice over the past ten years, but was unable to maintain it. Instead, she noted that her weight had fluctuated dramatically before she finally reached her present maximum of more than 200 pounds.

Sarah said, "I'd give anything to be back at my post-pregnancy weight of 140 pounds! I wish I'd never started that first diet, then maybe I wouldn't be in this mess. What made me think I was so fat back then?" Although weight loss was still important to Sarah, she was more interested in losing her weight-loss obsession and preventing further weight gain.

### Initial-Session Journal Entry:

I am *very* frustrated! I have tried so many fad diets and I'm sick of pills and calorie counting and all that stuff. I have been on the "diet roller coaster" for most of my adult life. I have lost and regained weight more times than I can count. My metabolism seems so messed up now, it's a wonder I have the strength to get out of bed in the morning. I'm obsessed with food/weight/exercise and I am so miserable. It affects my personal relationships, work, social life. All I think about is food and diets. I am so miserable. I have read every weight-loss book I can get my hands on. I am so desperate now and still just want to get this weight off!

I realize I have a big problem and it's more than the number on the scale. I know I need to stop all of this diet craziness, but I'm afraid of what will happen to my body if I stop trying to lose weight. I guess I have to take a chance, because I know that another diet is not the answer. I hope this works . . .

### *Initial Steps on the Path:*

My primary focus with Sarah was increasing her awareness of *why* she was eating, as well as *what* she was choosing to eat. Sarah discovered that she ate most of the time for emotional reasons, estimating a distribution of 80 percent emotional desire, 20 percent physical desire and 0 percent physical need. She claimed to be "totally out of touch" with her body's true hunger, and noted that she made her food choices based on whatever she craved (labeling these choices as "bad") or what she perceived to be healthy (labeling these choices as "good").

We discussed ways to reframe her "good/bad" thinking, and established some boundaries to help reduce her emotional eating tendencies. Rather than "beating herself up" for overeating, Sarah began to use each eating experience as an opportunity to discover the type and amount of food that would best satisfy her true hunger.

I also worked with Sarah to manage her emotions, rather than using food as a means of coping. Applying these same concepts to exercise, Sarah began to experiment with the type and amount of exercise that her body needed, instead of viewing exercise as an obligation. She began taking walks on a regular basis, and also incorporated strength training to help rebuild the lean body mass she'd lost during her years of dieting.

### Midway-Session Journal Entry:

It's been hard to let go of the "diet mentality." I keep telling myself what I "should" eat, and then I hear that "should" voice and I know that it's not my intuition. But where is my intuition? It still seems hard to hear. I feel like I need more structure. I know I just need to get used to not having so much structure. The structure is what has blocked my intuition, but without the structure I feel like I'll just eat everything in sight. Although, as I think about it, I really haven't done that. I can actually eat some of my old "forbidden foods" without overeating them. I suppose that's a victory!

I guess I'm just frustrated, because I started to lose weight, but now it seems like I have reached a plateau. I know weight is not supposed to be the important thing, but it was feeling good to lose some of this weight and I am frustrated that it seems to have stopped. So, what are my options here? I can keep going with this, trusting my body to end up at the weight that's right for me, or I can go back and try to lose the weight intentionally. But that's right back where I started—again. I don't want to go back there . . .

### Midway Steps on the Path:

Sarah's progress during the first two months involved *internal* changes, resulting in freedom from her obsessive weight loss focus. However, as Sarah's body began to decrease in size in response to her internal changes, she became attached again to the outcome of weight loss. She liked the experience of her clothes getting looser and she wanted this to continue. Although she dropped two dress sizes, she became frustrated when her weight stabilized here, because it was still a larger size than she wanted to be. She began to doubt herself and the process of Intuitive Self-Care.

At this point, I worked with Sarah to take the focus away from weight loss as her goal. We worked on going more deeply into her inner experience, emphasizing how she felt *in* her body. As a result, Sarah discovered that she in fact felt much better *inside* than she had in years. We reviewed her progress in learning *why* she was eating, and Sarah discovered that she had shifted to 30 percent emotional desire, 20 percent physical desire, and 50 percent physical need. With the awareness of her *internal* improvements, Sarah was more accepting of the *external* changes that her body was making. As we explored some of her career and relationship goals, Sarah began to realize that her identity was much more than her weight, and that success involved much more than weight loss.

### *Concluding-Session Journal Entry:*

I have really been LIVING lately! I can see my body as a beautiful instrument, capable of serving and enhancing my life in countless ways, rather than as a superficial object for others' viewing pleasure. You have NO idea what a milestone this is for me, and how it has freed me in my career and personal life. The ACT AS IF philosophy has helped me to realize that what I really want is to be the best ME that I can be.

I feel beautiful, lovable, and strong. It's amazing, I have made these things my goals, and they have happened! And, weight loss is taking care of itself. I feel so amazingly powerful now that I am free from the tremendously huge "weight" of diet obsession and compulsion. I am so happy, I have my life and my Self back again . . .

***Final Steps on the Path:***
After nine months, Sarah reported more progress in understanding the reasons *why* she ate, noting that she felt free of her emotional attachment to food. Although she did drop another dress size (ending up at a size 22), she stated that her real victory was no longer feeling like a slave to food and to the number on the bathroom scale. We reviewed the strategies that Sarah found to be most helpful, and discussed her plans to keep practicing these on a regular basis. I encouraged Sarah to continue her application of the concepts of Intuitive Self-Care to all areas of her life.

## Escapist Eric

At 6'0" and 320 pounds, Eric stated that he really didn't mind his large size, and was starting to accept that he'd be "fat forever." He started sessions with me at the prompting of his wife, who was worried about his health. His physician also expressed concern, indicating that Eric had high blood pressure and was a borderline diabetic. However, Eric was resistant to any kind of "weight loss program," since he had tried several in the past and did not like adhering to their rigid structure.

Eric owned a delicatessen, and noted that he tended to eat frequent "small meals" consisting of samples of the various meats and cheeses. He was on his feet most hours of the day and did a fair amount of lifting heavy items at work, but admitted that this was his only "exercise."

### *Initial-Session Journal Entry:*

I've pretty much given up trying to lose weight. Nothing has ever worked. I don't eat much, but I also don't exercise much. I know I don't have a slow metabolism or anything, but I can't seem to lose any weight, so maybe I'm just going to be fat forever. People talk a lot about being "fat and happy." Well, I'm fat. And I pretend to be happy. I'm just trying to get used to being a big size.

But my wife is concerned about me being this overweight. I get so out of breath just climbing a flight of stairs, she's afraid I'll have a heart attack one of these days. And my doctor says I should lose some weight, or at least get out and start an exercise program. Everybody else thinks I should do something about my weight. But I've tried. Nothing has worked. I'm tired of trying so hard . . .

### *Initial Steps on the Path:*

Eric had become extremely complacent. My primary focus with him was to enhance his awareness of the messages his body was sending him about his eating and exercise choices. It was as if Eric's "feedback loop" was broken, offering him no awareness of the negative consequences of his behaviors. Eric realized that he ate primarily out of physical desire, unaware that he actually nibbled all day long on the food that was always available at his deli. He began to ask, "Why am I reaching for food?" and stopped eating if his answer was "Because it's there."

In addition, I encouraged Eric to experiment with new types

of foods instead of always eating what he had on hand at work. Because Eric had little familiarity with safe fitness guidelines and was in poor physical condition, I referred him to a personal trainer to help him incorporate of beginner-level fitness activities into his life.

### *Midway-Session Journal Entry:*

It seems like there are so many changes to make. Too many. So, I'm just trying a little at a time. Each week I pick one change to focus on. Last week I decided to eat vegetables. I always hated vegetables, but I'm trying to find ones I do like to add some variety to what I eat. This week, I've been paying more attention to why I eat. Most of the time it's just because it's there. I used to grab handfuls of candy and other snacks that are available at work. It was an automatic habit. Now, I'm eating less, as a conscious choice.

Next week, I set up a time to meet with a personal trainer. I realize that I need help to get a basic fitness program going. I am definitely dropping in size, and that feels good. I can actually button the top button of my shirts again! So far, this is a lot better than any diet or weight loss plan I've tried. There are a lot of changes to make, but I like the freedom to choose what works for me. I like being able to go at my own pace . . .

### *Midway Steps on the Path:*

We continued to focus on enhancing Eric's awareness of *why, what,* and *how much* he was eating. After about four months, Eric noted that he was eating 75 to 100 percent of the time for physical need, and 0 to 25 percent of the time for physical desire. He noted that it was challenging to overcome his habit of sampling food at work, but he described feeling so much better since he was no longer overfeeding his body. This positive benefit outweighed his desire to snack. Eric's success was primarily due to his willingness to experiment—to try giving up old, unhelpful eating and exercise patterns and to replace them with new, nurturing ones.

### Concluding-Session Journal Entry:

What a difference! I feel so much better in my body now. And to think I would have "settled" to be "fat forever." My body size is still large, but I don't consider myself "fat" any more. I feel "big and healthy." My doctor is amazed at the changes I've made. My weight and cholesterol levels have both dropped. I ran into someone I hadn't seen in a few years, and he didn't recognize me! People are always asking me how I lost the weight, and I tell them I took the focus off the weight and put it on my health.

I'm more aware now of my food choices, and it feels good to eat more than just junk food all the time. Getting a regular fitness program going has been life-changing. I'm still working with that trainer, and I plan to keep doing it. The consistency feels good. If I'd known this is how things would turn out, I'd have done this a long time ago . . .

### Final Steps on the Path:

We concluded our sessions after about six months. Eric was pleased with his weight loss, but he described *internal factors* as his primary motivators to continue with the changes he had made. Specifically, he noted increased energy, improved blood chemistry, and an overall sense of inner balance. We reviewed the strategies that were working for Eric, and discussed an ongoing action plan.

## Busy Beth

Beth initiated sessions with me due to a sense that for the past several months "something just was not right," and her doctor could find no medical cause for her symptoms. A divorced forty-two-year-old, she complained of chronic fatigue, and a lack of motivation on the job or to fulfill other obligations. Beth expressed extreme irritation when others needed something from her—a behavior not characteristic of her nature. She indicated that, in general, she had always had a giving spirit and was concerned by her recent lack of generosity. She described her demanding job as a social worker, and how she was barely able to keep up with what was expected of her.

At 5'8" and 120 pounds, Beth appeared slim but had poor muscle tone. For breakfast, she tended to stop by a local coffee shop for a donut and coffee. Lunch was usually some kind of fast food, or snacks from a vending machine at work. For dinner, she typically popped a frozen meal into the microwave.

With the exception of going dancing about once a week, Beth did not participate in any fitness activities. She expressed interest in changing her eating and exercise habits, but felt no motivation to follow through. She noted a pattern of staying up late at night to watch television, often not turning out the light until 1 A.M. She described a feeling of dread in the morning as her alarm clock went off, and a lethargy that lasted all day. On weekends, although she often slept until noon, she indicated feeling the same lethargy throughout the day.

### Initial-Session Journal Entry:

I'm just not feeling my best lately. I seem to be getting sick more easily, and I know I'm not really taking good care of myself. I'm just not real motivated to change. I've got a lot going on in my life, and when I get home from work I just don't feel like working out. Maybe that's an excuse, I don't know. Maybe I'm afraid I'll get compulsive with it? No, I guess it's just not a priority. I feel like I should exercise more and eat better though, so how do I get that motivation back? I really wouldn't care about any of this, but I just haven't been feeling good. I've got too much to do in my life to feel this crappy. So, I hope something can change . . .

### Initial Steps on the Path:

Working in a helping profession, Beth was constantly giving to others at the expense of herself. She had no energy left to nurture her own body, mind, and soul. Beth focused intensely on what she "should do"—both for others and herself. However, she resisted these demands, berated herself for not following through, felt guilty, and then dictated what she "should do" all over again. We explored ways to end this exhausting cycle, shifting from outer-directed "shoulds" to inner-directed "needs." We worked on tuning in to the messages from her body, mind, and soul, and how she could change her schedule to honor her true needs.

### Midway-Session Journal Entry:

Well, I'm still not feeling really motivated. I know what I should do, but I just don't seem able to do it. Maybe that's the problem. I'm telling myself I should do it instead of letting it be an internal process. Oh, this is going to take more time than I wanted! Or maybe that's a good thing. I'm starting to realize that I haven't made myself much of a priority lately. I come last. Maybe I can try an experiment and put some of my own needs first for a change . . .

### Midway Steps on the Path:

Beth discovered that her "should" voice had an iron grip on her. With practice over the next six months, Beth was able to hear her own intuitive voice more clearly. She found it helpful to affirm that she deserved to make positive changes and that it was OK to take care of herself first. Writing in her journal also helped Beth to turn up the volume of her soul's wisdom. By reviewing her entries, she could see when she was "shoulding" herself versus when her intuition was guiding her actions. Tuning in more deeply to her body's needs allowed Beth to make an inner commitment to improving her eating habits and fitness level.

### Concluding-Session Journal Entry:

I feel like I have a new life! The biggest change was giving time to myself every morning. Now my first appointment in my daytimer is the one with ME. I take time to write in my journal every day, and this helps me to monitor my stress levels. Also, I've "allocated the opportunity to be active" each morning. Getting back into fitness has been great. I had forgotten how good it feels! My motivation now is to keep feeling good. I know there was a part of me that was resisting a fitness plan because I didn't want to go overboard. But I compromised my fitness in the process. I'm glad I found the right balance for me . . .

### Final Steps on the Path:

After about six months, Beth and I concluded our sessions. We reviewed the strategies that she was using to keep in touch with her intuition. I encouraged Beth to continue to experiment with the type and amount of exercise that was best for her specific needs.

*What are some of your concerns about the journey of freedom? What did you learn through your archetype's perspective? Try writing in your journal about any fears and doubts that you may have. See if the voice of your soul offers you its wisdom about how to proceed. Can you trust the process and begin your journey of freedom?*

# Section III

~ ~

# Soulful Strategies

# feed your
# hungry soul

During your previous attempts to control your weight, you may have noticed an insatiable hunger that binge eating could not satisfy nor starvation deny. That's because this "hunger" is from your soul. Your soul has been heavily burdened by all of your dieter's games—and the more nourishment you provide for it, the lighter and freer it will become. *You lose the weight from your soul by feeding your soul.*

But what is your soul "hungry" for? *Your attention.* Your soul is "hungry" for you to listen to its voice, the guidance of your intuition. Your soul is "hungry" for you to shift from being outer-guided to being inner-guided, learning to live your life from the inside out. Your soul is "hungry" for you to be your spiritually conscious Self, whole and complete as a soul/mind/body. *Your soul is "hungry" for you to practice Intuitive Self-Care.*

The central theme of Intuitive Self-Care is to "live from your soul"—to see, think, feel, act and be from your spiritual consciousness. There are five principles that define how you can do this:

- Love your Self

- Be true to your Self

- Express your Self

- Give to your Self

- Believe in your Self

Think of these principles as the "nourishment for your soul," like a five-course meal beginning with an "appetizer" and ending with "dessert." Just as the body needs food to survive, the soul needs its own kind of nourishment to grow and to be effective in guiding your life. This nourishment is anything that enhances your ability to listen to and act on your own intuitive wisdom. *Follow this spiritual "diet" and offer your soul the nourishment that it needs.*

I learned these five principles on my own journey of freedom, and I began using them as affirmations. I wrote them in my journal every day, and then reflected on how I could apply them in my life. Each day I developed a deeper understanding of these principles, and ultimately discovered that their application went far beyond the resolution of weight issues. These five principles are universal; they will help solve not only weight problems but also other "weighty issues" in your life. They teach the concept that "success is an inside job," and help you apply intuitive wisdom to improve relationships, enhance career satisfaction, and achieve other goals in your personal and professional lives. *Apply these five principles to your life, and watch your entire life change.*

## BREADCRUMBS ALONG THE JOURNEY

Since the five principles are so significant, many people have asked how I learned them. Did I read them in a deeply profound piece of literature? Did I hear them from a wise and insightful sage on a remote mountaintop? Or did I just randomly stumble upon them one day in a conversation with a complete stranger? There definitely were messengers involved—but not a book, a sage, or a stranger. The messengers were unique, because they happened to be my pets: a parakeet, a young kitten, and an older kitten (now my cat). Messengers can take many forms—authors, therapists, friends, acquaintances, strangers—and even other kinds of life such as nature or animals.

Any soul can be a messenger. We receive messages all the time, like breadcrumbs along our path, showing us the way. These breadcrumbs serve as markers, reminding us where we've been. And they serve as guideposts, pointing out the direction in which we should proceed. The trick is to be open to the messengers and their messages. It's up to each of us to find those breadcrumbs on our path, to pay attention to the messages that can help us on our journey.

## The Gift of Wings

I got Peppy, my parakeet, at a time when my eating and weight problems were at their worst. But Peppy saw me through those troubled times. The three phrases that Peppy said over and over were his messages to me. First, he'd sit and gaze at himself in a little mirror he had in his cage. "I love you, I love you, I love you," he'd repeat. He'd also say "Gimme a kiss," while tapping his beak against his image in the mirror and making a kissing noise. The last thing I was able to do at that time in my life was look in the mirror and say "I love you" to myself! I could barely stand to look at myself in the mirror, and there was no way I'd send any affection toward myself as Peppy did with his kisses. But that's exactly what I needed to do: love my soul, mind, and body. "Love your Self," he was trying to say.

The third message Peppy had for me was a question. When I first brought Peppy home, his wings had been clipped, which is standard procedure for caged birds. However, I wanted Peppy to know the joy of freedom, so I let his wings grow back and I kept the door to his cage open so that he could fly around my apartment. Sometimes, in the midst of my binges and purges, Peppy would fly over to me, sit on my shoulder, and say "What are ya doin'?" "Go away," I'd yell back at him, and shrug my shoulder to make him leave. Then he'd usually fly around the apartment, chirping away in freedom and bliss, while I continued with my eating frenzy. Peppy had a powerful message for me through his words and example; what I needed to do was *listen*. I needed to ask myself exactly what I was doing by stuffing my body with food and ignoring my true needs. He was showing me the alternative—that I too could fly freely, if I just let my own wings grow back so I could escape the cage I'd built around myself. I needed to be true to my soul, mind, and body. "Be true to your Self," he was trying to say.

## An Angel on a Misty Morning

Misty was a typical playful kitten, and he reminded me of the importance of experiencing joy in my own life. But Misty also taught me about experiencing pain as well. A few weeks after I brought Misty home from a stray cat's litter, he started to have brief seizures during which his entire body would shake for a few seconds. No medical cause was ever identified for Misty's seizures. Symbolically, Misty was giving me a warning of what could happen to me. His seizures were analogous to a "nervous breakdown"—a possibility for me if I didn't manage my emotions. I had learned strategies to acknowledge my feelings, but I still tended to stuff my emotions away, especially those I didn't like. It was easier to express the "positive" feelings, but I needed to continue to openly express *all* feelings, keeping the balance of my soul, mind, and body. Misty was showing me the potential consequences if I didn't. "Express your Self," he was trying to say.

Misty also gave me another message. I had been living at my Freedom point for a period of a few months, but I was starting to take my healing for granted. I figured I'd reached that place of "complete recovery" that my therapist always talked about. I didn't realize the importance of *maintaining* my healing practices in order to maintain my freedom. I was becoming complacent. I'd eat whenever I got around to it, whatever was available, no longer taking care to give my body what it really needed when it needed it. Similarly, I'd work out if there was time, without checking in with my body about its true needs for fitness. I'd squeeze in journaling around my other daily activities, and began to skip entries. I was feeling stressed, I was overeating and underexercising, and my body was putting on weight as a result.

Meanwhile, Misty's seizures continued. It was as if the chaos in my life was being mirrored by his behavior. But there was a difference between Misty and me. My life felt chaotic all the time, whereas Misty, in between his seizures, seemed to still be enjoying his life. I would see him napping, bathing, eating, or playing. Misty reminded me of how important it is for me to nourish my soul, mind, and body, especially in the midst of chaos. "Give to your Self," he was trying to say.

## Going the Extra Mile

On a visit to Northern Michigan, while out for a run on a back-country road, I noticed an animal walking in the road up ahead. At first glance, it appeared to be a small raccoon. As I neared, I realized it was a black, tan, and white kitten! She meowed and ran toward me, as if to say "It's about time you showed up!" I stopped and picked her up, and she purred immediately. I looked around for other kittens or the mother cat, but none was in sight. I put her down, saying "Find your mom, kitty," and I started to run again. I had about a mile left to go, and she followed me. I would stop periodically to pick her up, afraid she'd give herself a heart attack running with me so far. But when I'd put her down with a firm "Go home, kitty," and start running again, she continued to follow me.

That kitten ran with me the whole mile—hence her name, Miler. It seemed she had found her home with me. I can only imagine how difficult it was for Miler to run that entire mile. Her example was reminding me that I could go the distance, too. Many times since then I have faced situations that seemed overwhelming, but then I remember that I'm not doing anything alone any more. I always have my soul's guidance. Just as I led Miler through her difficult run, my soul is always leading me on that extra mile. "Believe in your Self," she was trying to say.

## THE "DIET" TO NOURISH YOUR SOUL

The breadcrumbs left on my path by Peppy, Misty, and Miler were "food for my soul," providing me with the five principles that continue to enhance my life. But these breadcrumbs have been left for you as well. You can take their messages and apply them to your life. The five principles are the "diet" to nourish your hungry soul, serving to enhance the connection among your soul, mind, and body. *Love your Self. Be true to your Self. Express your Self. Give to your Self. Believe in your Self.*

## To Whet Your Appetite—Love Your Self

Loving your Self is "seeing with your soul," seeing from the inside out. How does your soul "see" your body? Your mind? The world around you? Loving your Self is loving your whole Self, as a soul/mind/body. Loving your Self is honoring your soul as your core essence. Loving your Self is honoring your mind and its thoughts and feelings as unique expressions of your soul. Loving your Self is honoring your body as the unique vessel your soul has chosen in which to live and experience the world.

Loving your Self is a genuine, soulful love for your entire being, conveying a sense of wholeness. It is impossible to love only parts of yourself, such as just your mind but not your body, or just your eyes but not your thighs. You are a whole being, and your soul's love is for the whole of you. If you dislike any part you dislike the whole. Your soul sees only the whole of you, not separate parts. Your soul invites you to see yourself as it sees you, a whole being. Your soul invites you to feel the love it feels for you, regardless of factors such as size, shape, intelligence, or finances. Loving your Self is unconditional love, a love that is not contingent on circumstances.

As you explore the concept of loving your Self, you may worry that you'll become narcissistic. However, narcissism is self-obsession, not Self-love. Narcissism can occur if you are an outer-guided world/mind/body self, obsessed with making your body fit the world's standards. Your body can literally be the object of your worship, leading you to do anything to get it to fit that ideal: weight loss, body building, plastic surgery—anything to enhance your outward appearance. But of course you'll never look quite good enough, and you'll remain stuck in your narcissistic quest.

Because our society places such an emphasis on looks, is it any wonder that we can become narcissistic? We are bombarded with messages about how our bodies "should look," and if we don't feel we measure up, we berate ourselves. The standards of beauty that we impose on ourselves merely fuel our desire to change our bodies, get rid of cellulite, burn fat, shed pounds, tone muscles, tuck tummies, and so on. The body that we have never seems "good enough." But if you were on a desert island where no one else was around, and there were no beauty magazines to compare yourself to, how would you feel about your body? You would have no reason to criticize it or to obsess over making it "better."

Instead, we judge, evaluate, criticize, and berate our bodies for not measuring up to some unattainable standard we have set for ourselves. Rather than honoring our own body's unique shape and size, we try to make it conform to society's ideals. We try to mold our bodies into something that is not natural, because we have bought the lie that we are not already good enough.

Perhaps your body has accumulated a few extra pounds—or many. Or perhaps your body is too thin. Whatever the case, your body is what it is today. This is the only body you have right now. You have two choices at this moment: Hate your body or love your Self. Which do you choose?

You may be thinking, "But if I love my Self, then I'll be fat forever!" No. If you love your Self, then you open the door for miracles to happen. Because when you love your Self, you are loving your soul, mind, and body. Loving your Self reconnects you with your soul's wisdom, so you can practice Intuitive Self-Care. However, if you hate your body, the opposite will happen.

Think about it. If you had a friend who yelled at you and told you how fat and ugly you are, and another friend who told you how wonderful you are, which one would you want to listen to? Which one would motivate you? Your soul wants to help you, if you will let it. Your soul wants to show you yourself from its perspective.

When you learn to see with your soul, you are aligning your perception of yourself, others, and the world around you with your spiritual essence. We tend to see with the body's eyes, but the key is to see with the soul's eyes. Your soul appreciates everything exactly as it is in each moment. When you see with your soul, you see beyond any perceived limitations. You see the perfection of everything exactly as it is. There is no judgment.

Whenever you hear criticism, you are seeing with your body's eyes, not with your soul. When you see with your soul, you are letting your soul experience what is. You do not just observe, you experience. With the body's eyes you might comment, "Oh, look at that beautiful sunset!" But when you see with your soul, you really feel the beauty at a much deeper level of appreciation and understanding. When you see a sunset from your soul's perspective, you internalize it, as if the sunset were radiating throughout your entire being.

When you see your body with your soul's eyes, you are not only looking at your body, you are also enjoying the experience of *being in* your body. What does it feel like to have the incredible body that you have? Your body is your soul's eyes, arms, legs, feet, and hands; your soul needs your body to live. Your body is part of your soul's unique experience of you. Everyone's body is different, and the soul values and appreciates these differences. Seeing with your soul, you can admire external beauty in others' bodies, without envy. You can feel a connection with others, instead of a separation. You can enjoy a sense of completion, rather than a sense of lack. With Self-love, you can finally be happy.

Self-love is the path of happiness because, in general, what makes us unhappy is our own critical perception of ourselves (and our life situations). You have everything you need in this moment to be absolutely happy. It is only your observation that something is missing or not good enough that is making you unhappy. The wonderful thing about happiness is that it builds on itself. Once you are grateful and appreciative of all you have, you will find that more will come your way.

## The Main Course—Be True to Your Self

Being true to your Self is "thinking with your soul," thinking from the inside out. This involves holding in your mind the thoughts that your soul would have you think. Being true to your Self is listening to and following the voice of your soul, as it guides you with eating, exercise, relationships, career, and all areas of your life.

Being true to your Self is honoring your intuition, and applying its wisdom by living in wholeness as a soul/mind/body. This is a life of integrity—every thought you think and every response to your thoughts is congruent with your core essence. Being true to your Self is using your soul's wisdom in all of your decision-making. From your soul's perspective, what choices are healthy for your body? Healthy for your mind? Healthy for your life?

Being true to your Self is living a truly healthy life as an expression of your soul's wisdom. The key is to align your mind with your soul, to think from the inside. We tend to think from the outside, with the mind aligned with the world. This is the "traditional" way to think: intellectual, logical, and fact-oriented. But when you think with your soul, it's very intuitive, insightful, and introspective. Can you relate to your mind's operating in both these ways? In any moment, you can choose to "think with your soul" or to "think with the world." You can listen to your intuition or you can follow the advice of others. You can trust your own inner wisdom or you can look outside yourself for society's perspectives. The choice to be inner-guided or outer-guided is always there.

And, with every choice, there are consequences. The soul's choices always bring peace, while the world's choices always bring conflict, like weight problems and eating disorders, or other symptoms such as stress, anxiety, depression. Symptoms are messengers, showing the effects of the choices you make, giving you the opportunity to ask, "Is this what I choose for my soul to experience?" You are always free to choose again. You can go more deeply within yourself to access the thoughts your soul would have you hear. You can apply your soul's wisdom in your decision making. You can use your soul's guidance to change your life.

The next time you make a decision, ask, "Is this my soul's voice or the world's voice guiding my choice right now?" Be aware. Make conscious choices. You don't have to ignore everything that others say, or isolate yourself from the voices of the world. You just need to be aware of these messages, and discern whether or not they are congruent with the voice of your soul. Notice the messages that you get from the world, and process them in an intuitive way. Take the information that you are given from other people and the world around you, and run it through your own internal filter. Check in with yourself and ask, "Does this fit for me? Does this have real meaning to me?" Many people hear guidelines about what we "should eat," and these are fine to experiment with. But take the process from the world's view to your soul's perspective. Think with your soul, not with the rules. What does your soul say about nutrition guidelines? Which ones is your soul telling you to try?

When you are outer-guided, you are looking to get something—approval, praise, money, weight loss. When you are inner-guided and true to your Self, you are looking to give something— your passion, unique talents and abilities, nutrition and health to your body. Being true to your Self does not mean that you withdraw from the world; rather, it allows you to be in the world in a way that has real meaning. It's a way to *give to* rather than *get from.*

Sometimes the voices of other souls can help you hear the voice of your own soul more effectively. However, sometimes others try to impose their own will upon you, rather than helping you to discover yours. You need to recognize the difference. It's a little bit like solving a puzzle—the puzzle of your life. Some people will help you turn over the pieces you couldn't see, or help you find a piece that was missing, enhancing your ability to piece together your life and be true to your Self. However, others will take pieces away from your puzzle and they'll throw in some pieces from *their* puzzle. Being true to your Self is recognizing this before it happens, maintaining your boundaries as it happens, and avoiding being taken in by these situations in the future. Being true to your Self is connecting with the people and situations instead that enhance your ability to solve your puzzle, that help you go within yourself to find your own unique solutions.

Any time you detect the word "should" in your language, it's a sign that you are thinking with the world. "Should" is rooted in either the past (guilt) or the future (worry), as in "I should work out because I feel guilty that I didn't do it yesterday," or "I should skip lunch to cut back on calories because otherwise I'll worry too much when I'm out for dinner later." To shift from the world to the soul, change from "should" to "choose." Instead of saying "I really *should* do x, y, z," ask "What do I *choose* to do?" This question takes you within, to access your soul's wisdom. "Choice" keeps you in the present, with what you need right now. In this moment, what do you choose? What is your soul telling you that you need? If you could let go of your past regrets (because the past is over) and future worries (because the future isn't here), what does the present reveal to you? *Be here now.* If you made every decision based on your present needs, being true to your Self in each moment, then you'd never have guilt and you'd never have to worry!

It can be scary at first to be true to your Self and think with your soul. This is because you have been taught that answers are found outside of you, not within. You may wonder whether you can really trust your intuitive wisdom. But remember, your soul's voice is really your link with God, a Higher Power, Universal Intelligence, or whatever you choose to call it. If you choose to ignore your soul's voice and listen to the world instead, it's like you're saying "No, sorry God, I don't trust you, I know more than you do, I think I'll just keep doing it my way." In contrast, thinking with your soul is operating in union with your spiritual design. When people say "Let go and let God," they are letting go of their own personal, outer-guided way of handling things, and tuning in to their spiritual, inner-guided solutions. Being true to your Self is releasing control and opening up to wisdom.

You may be so convinced that others know more than you do that you forget to look *inside* yourself for the answers you seek. Diets and weight-loss plans fail because they take you further and further away from your own wisdom. After dieting for years, you may not even be aware of the signals that your body sends you as guidance. You might not know what hunger and fullness are any more. You can become fearful of trusting your body, because you may be concerned that you will not reach the weight-loss goals you have in mind. You fear that you will "get fat" if you eat what you seem to be truly hungry for, or if you listen to your body when it needs a break from activity.

However, as evidenced by the case studies and clients' testimonials in this book, it is this inner wisdom that your body naturally possesses that will *guide you to freedom* from your weight problem. Your body knows the amount of food and type of food that is right for you. Your body also knows the amount and type of activity that is best for you at different points in time. If you learn to listen to this inner wisdom, and to trust your body, you will find that your body will gravitate to the weight that is right for you.

Being true to your Self is the path of health because, in general, what makes us unhealthy is our own choice to ignore our inner wisdom. This inner wisdom, the voice of the soul, guides the health of the mind and body. Honoring intuition facilitates the process of a whole, healthy life. You have everything you need in this moment to be truly healthy. It is only your choice to align your mind with the world's dictates of how you "should" live that is making you unhealthy. The healthier your attitude becomes, the healthier you will become as your whole Self.

## On the Side—Express Your Self

Expressing your Self is "feeling with your soul," feeling from the inside out. This involves letting your emotions be experienced from your soul's perspective. Expressing your Self is honoring all of your feelings, and letting your soul reveal the process of moving through them as part of your life experience. Your soul knows a deeper purpose in your emotions, and it will guide you in discovering this. Expressing your Self is letting your emotions flow and be in balance. You enjoy the highs without attachment, and you honor the lows without resistance. As an emotion surfaces, your soul guides you to feel it, experience it, learn from it, and release it. Expressing your Self is honoring your emotions as part of your soul's unique experience living as you in the world.

This is completely contrary to what we are taught about emotions. From childhood we learn things like "Little girls are sugar and spice," and "Children should be seen and not heard," which send the message that it's not acceptable to express how we feel. "Crying is a sign of weakness," and "Keep your chin up and be strong," are pervasive messages that we carry into adulthood. Then there are the messages of pop culture, such as "Don't worry, be happy," and "Just put on a happy face." Major industries are built around the avoidance of certain emotions and the attainment of others, such as pharmaceutical companies whose advertisements seem to say "Pop a pill, get rid of your depression, and live happily ever after."

Is it any wonder that we view some feelings as "good" and others as "bad," and that we strive to find and hold onto the "good" feelings while trying to eliminate and avoid the "bad" ones? Depression, anxiety, anger, and fear are typically labeled "bad" emotions. We're told to "just get over things," and as a result we stuff those emotions inside. Or we try to logic our way through our feelings, telling ourselves how irrational it is to feel those "bad" emotions. For example, if we feel afraid of something, we make a list of reasons why we really shouldn't feel that way. We gather evidence in an attempt to shut down the fear. We tell ourselves "Just do it!" but the fear inside is still screaming, "Please don't!"

Those "bad" emotions have a message for us, if we'd just take the time to listen. And, until we do listen, the emotions—although unacknowledged—are still there, accumulating inside of us. They build up, and are often released in a burst of intense emotion such as a violent rage or a nervous breakdown. In her book *Women's Bodies, Women's Wisdom,* Dr. Christiane Northrup indicates that unexpressed emotions are stored in our bodies and can express themselves as physical symptoms such as headaches, colds, aches, pains, abnormal growths, or even cancer. Eating disorders are a classic example of this, with restrictive eating, binge eating, and purging—all symptoms that reflect the body's way to cope with and attempt to release unexpressed emotions. Such symptoms are the soul's way of utilizing the body to get our attention, to guide us in changing the way we handle our emotions.

We want the "good" without the "bad," the "ups" without the "downs," and society seems to promise we can have it this way. But that's a myth. While it may seem appealing to focus only on the "good" emotions, it's important to realize that life is a balance of good and bad. What makes our good times even better is experiencing the bad ones. The fullness of our emotions adds richness and depth to our lives. We need to let go of the stereotypes we have formed about the "bad" emotions and learn to let them flow. We need to learn what they are here to teach us. This means undoing the messages you have learned about emotions, and opening up to your intuitive guidance about them.

Emotions must be acknowledged. Think about a persistent door-to-door salesman, someone who keeps knocking on your door day after day. Your emotions are like that salesman, and if you just open the door and let the emotions in, they will stop bothering you. The salesman will go away once he has had the opportunity to share his sales pitch with you. Unlike the salesman, your emotions have nothing to sell you. They simply want their message to be heard. Like the tides of the ocean, we need to let our emotions ebb and flow, come and go. Sometimes the tide comes in with joy. Sometimes it recedes with sadness. Then it comes in again with contentment. Then it pulls back again with anger. When we stop resisting the emotions and let them flow, a natural balance results.

The yin and yang symbols from ancient Chinese philosophy

represent the male and female principles of the universe, and reflect the concept of balance. These symbols are often depicted as a circle that is half black and half white. The black and white halves swirl into each other, illustrating the interconnectedness of male and female energies, and of darkness and light. Each half also contains a small circle of the opposite color within it—white within black, black within white—the seed of the other within itself. The same is true of our emotions. Those dark emotions contain the seed of light. Somewhere amidst depression, anxiety, and anger is a positive element just waiting to surface.

Balance is not about "getting rid of" the dark emotions. It is about converting them into a usable form. A metaphor of this process is the ancient belief in alchemy, which posited the transmutation of base metals into gold. We need to be "emotional alchemists," transforming dark emotions into light. Another illustration of this process is based on the common adage, "When life gives you lemons, make lemonade." Turn sour situations into sweet opportunities. Depression in and of itself may not seem desirable. However, the outcome of experiencing and moving through depression often offers the opportunity for deep insights, healing, and growth. Many authors, artists, scientists, and others describe having their most profound insights during or following periods of intense dark emotions.

This transformation from darkness into light occurs by moving through the emotions, by feeling them fully. In his book *Care of the Soul,* Thomas Moore suggests that we have rooms in our house or places in our garden where we can retreat to *be with* those dark emotions. At first, this may seem very unappealing: Why would one *want* to be depressed? But you are *not* your emotions. The essential thing to learn is to *be with* your emotions, not *be of* them. Stay centered as a soul/mind/body, and experience your emotions without becoming your emotions. Instead of saying "I *am* depressed," say "I *feel* depressed." Notice the difference?

Expressing your Self is the path of balance because, in general, what makes us unbalanced is our own refusal to feel the fullness of all our emotions. Balance is restored and maintained by using the soul's wisdom to experience the depth of both dark and light emotions.

## For Your Refreshment—Give to Your Self

Giving to your Self is "acting with your soul," acting from the inside out. This involves taking the actions in your life that your soul would have you do. Giving to your Self is about following through on what you know you need to do to be true to your Self. It's changing your priorities so that you are spending time on what's really important. Giving to your Self is about practicing Intuitive Self-Care in your everyday life, and letting the benefits that you experience extend outward to others.

From your soul's perspective, what actions are nourishing for your body? Nourishing for your mind? Nourishing for others and the world around you? Giving to your Self is about making win-win decisions, those which honor your soul and the souls in all of life. You actions bring peace to you and those around you. Giving to your Self is living in reverence of your soul's wisdom.

You may be concerned that giving to your Self is "selfish." But there is a difference between giving to your self as an outer-guided world/mind/body and giving to your Self as an inner-guided soul/mind/body. Selfishness is giving to the small self, the separate self, the world/mind/body self. Selfishness is taking action based on what you can *get from* the world, often at the expense of others. In contrast, think of giving to your Self as being Self-full, not selfish. Self-fullness is taking action based on what you can *give to* the world. Of course, the world includes others . . . and *you*. Giving to your Self is a way to "fill your Self up" so that you have more to give to others. Giving to your Self is honoring your needs as a soul/mind/body first, and then giving to others from your own reservoir filled with nourishment.

Think of your Self as a well. In order to gave water to others, you first have to get the well flowing. Once the well is overflowing, you can then share what you have with others. But you need to maintain the flow of your well, to be sure you are not giving away more than you have coming in. Otherwise, if you keep giving at the expense of your Self, your well will dry up. Giving to your Self is about *starting* the flow, *increasing* the flow, *sharing* the flow, and *maintaining* the flow of your own well. Giving to your Self is taking care of your own needs first, and then attending to others.

We usually learn this the other way around. We are taught to attend to others' needs first, and then our own. However, often we can end up giving to others but never taking care of ourselves. We give, but at the expense of the Self. This is often referred to as the "martyr syndrome." If you recognize this tendency in yourself, then it's important to realize that you cannot effectively give to others unless you attend to your own needs first. If you've ever flown on a commercial airplane, you are familiar with the flight attendant's information about changes in cabin air pressure. An oxygen mask will automatically drop, and the instruction is to "secure your own mask first before assisting others."

The same is true in our own lives. In a sense, we stifle our own breath by always giving to others first. We often "kill ourselves" in the process of trying to help others. There is nothing wrong with giving to others, but the key is to "secure your own mask first"—to fortify yourself first so you are better able to assist others.

When you are giving to your Self, it's as if you are making your body a home for your soul. But not just any home—you are making it a home that you love to be in and that you love to open up and share with others. Giving to your Self is about being "the best you that you can be." It's about following through on everything that you know you need to do to be true to your Self. It's setting new priorities and establishing new routines that make Intuitive Self-Care an inherent part of your life. It's making the most important commitment you will ever make—to your Self as a soul/mind/body.

As your happy, healthy, balanced, and peaceful Self, imagine the life you can live and the difference that you can make in the world. People often pray for their dreams to come true, and then sit back and wait for something to happen. But prayer is really designed to awaken our own intentions, motivating our own actions from within, as an inner-guided soul/mind/body. Giving to your Self is like becoming the answer to your own prayer. It's taking responsibility for your own life, and taking the action that your soul guides you to take, to make your own dreams come true.

This process of giving to your Self is what I call "re-parenting." It's giving your Self the nurturing that you really need, and perhaps never received enough of as a child. You can be the parent you always wished you had. During a conference I attended recently, eating-disorders therapists Dr. Mark Schwartz and Lisa Gilpern used the term "empathic attunement" to describe an appropriately sensitive and connected relationship between parent and child. When parents are properly attuned in an empathic manner to their child, they know when to touch or hold the child, and when to pull back. It's a bit like a dance, with partners coming together and moving apart in a congruent manner. However, when not properly attuned to the child, parents are not attentive when the child needs it, and/or they overstimulate the child when the child needs space.

As a therapist, I often serve the role of the "parent" for my clients, leaning toward them when they need more empathy, pulling away when I sense they need space. I am modeling for them how they can treat themselves in an empathically attuned way. Ultimately my clients become the "parent" for themselves, learning how to respond to their own needs appropriately.

More often than not, people have experienced improper empathic attunement during their formative years. Parents weren't there, either physically or emotionally, when we needed to be held and loved. Parents were there, perhaps in an overprotective or even invasive manner, when we needed more space. Does this mean we are destined for a life of trauma, dysfunction, and disease? Does this mean we all need years and years of psychotherapy to recover? No. It just means we can benefit from "re-parenting" ourselves, by giving ourselves the empathic attunement we need. We must learn how to dance with ourselves, responding to our own needs, being attentive and nurturing. And when we have had enough, then we can reach out and give to others.

I call this inner nurturing "going down and in." These are times of introspection and solitude, with heightened sensitivity to our own personal needs. Reaching out to the world, I call "going up and out." These are times of inspiration and connection with others, with heightened sensitivity to others' needs. We need to learn the dance steps for both, to learn the intricate patterns of the dance that work the best for our souls.

As you start giving to your Self, you may find that you will actually need to *give things up*. At first you may resist this concept, because it can feel like you'll be depriving yourself of something. However, rather than thinking about what you'll be *sacrificing*, think about what you'll be *getting*. For example, overeating, binge eating, purging, overexercising, restrictive eating, exercise and weight rituals can be your *attempt* to take care of yourself. These rituals are probably very familiar, and offer some type of temporary relief. However, these symptoms are not addressing your true needs.

Giving to your Self is about meeting your true needs. Giving to your Self means leaving behind old patterns that do not work effectively. Giving to your Self means replacing ineffective rituals with new routines that reflect Intuitive Self-Care. In that sense, it's not a sacrifice, it's a gift. With every action that you take, ask yourself: "Is this the gift that I choose to give my soul right now?"

You may be aware of some resistance in giving to your Self. Resistance is always a sign that the "voices of the world" are crowding your awareness. You are telling yourself either, "I really *shouldn't* do this" or "I really *should* do that." Both messages will create resistance to your taking the steps to meet your true needs. The "shouldn't voice" is related to a concept that somehow you don't deserve to take care of your needs. Where does this voice come from? Did someone say this to you in your past? Contrary to what you may have been told, you absolutely do deserve to be nurtured and loved. You are worthy, exactly as you are. Try saying the affirmation "I deserve!"

As for the "should voice," this is a sign that you are imposing an outer-guided goal upon yourself instead of an inner-guided one. Take your directions from within rather than from without. Get in tune with the actions that your soul wants for you. Let these surface and be expressed as, "I choose to do this as a gift for my soul."

Give to your Self at the pace that's right for you. There are no speed records to break here. You don't have to change your whole life in one day. Giving to your Self is about *what* you do and also *how* you do it. There is no one right way. Only your soul knows the process that is truly right for you. Give yourself permission to speed up or slow down as needed. Give yourself the flexibility to change your routines when they no longer work. Give yourself forgiveness for mistakes as you learn from them. Give yourself exactly what you need. Give to your Self and enjoy peace in this moment and every moment.

I say that the benefit of giving to your Self is peace. Not peace in terms of world peace, but an inner peace or serenity within you. Of course, if we each carried this kind of inner peace with us each day, world peace would automatically follow. When have you experienced complete and total inner peace? Many of my clients say they never have. Some say they have but only fleetingly. And a few say they have it all the time. *All the time.* What would it be like to enjoy eternal peace? I believe that it is possible. We don't have to come and go from that place of peace. We can carry it with us, wherever we go, whatever we do.

## Don't Forget Dessert—Believe in Your Self

Believing in your Self is "being with your soul," being from the inside out. It's a sense of total connection with your soul, a sense of wholeness, an ability to truly *be who you really are.* This carries with you wherever you are. Believing in your Self is knowing that you and your soul are in union, now and for all eternity. You have found the voice of your soul again, and you will never lose your connection with it. That's because you *are* it. You are your soul's voice. You are your soul's body. You are your soul's life. Believing in your Self is being who you were meant to be, as a congruent extension of your soul.

Believing in your Self is what opens you to ongoing success. It is an affirmation that says "I own my greatness!" When you believe in your Self, you are expressing gratitude for all the good that has already unfolded in yourself; you are also affirming the blessings that you currently enjoy, and inviting more success to come into your life. You are acknowledging your progress toward freedom from your food, weight, and body worries, and toward your other goals in life. You are celebrating the partnership that you have with your soul. As Dr. Wayne Dyer says in *Manifest Your Destiny,* living your dreams is a process of co-creation. You do not create success on your own. You co-create success in partnership with your soul.

Believing in your Self is being confident. Confidence is pointing your faith in the direction of your soul. In contrast, fear is merely faith pointed in the wrong direction. Fear is what happens when you "forget who you really are." Fear is an outer-guided perspective. Fear is a call for you to remember your soul, and to reclaim your inner-guided reality.

During one of my workshops, a participant shared an acronym she used for fear: *Forgetting Everything's All Right.* Believe in your Self and trust the process of your life as it unfolds. Know that you already have all the answers to your success within you.

It is helpful if you have others who also believe in you. At times, if your fears and doubts surface, these others can help you regain your confidence. These are the people who are climbing that mountain with you, reaching down to pull you up just when you think you can't climb any higher. They offer you new perspectives on succeeding with Intuitive Self-Care. Or they are climbing along beside you, supporting you as they go along. They offer you encouragement to continue with Intuitive Self-Care. The voices of their souls can help you to stay connected with the voice of your own soul. That's when you realize that we're all in this together. At some level, we're all connected. When one of us succeeds, we all succeed.

And then there are the times when it feels like you are completely alone. You don't have someone close by to cheer you on. You can't find that hand reaching down to pull you up. It seems like the darkness is closing in, and you don't know which way to turn. You wonder whether you'll ever be free of your food, weight, and body worries. You're feeling lost, and you just want someone to show you the way. And it's at times like these that you'll actually find the greatest guide of all—the guide that's always within you. You are never alone. The voice of your soul goes with you wherever you go. In the midst of the darkness you can always find the light within your Self. Just believe . . . in your Self.

*What does each of these five principles mean to you? How can you apply them to your own life? What other messages have you received that are like breadcrumbs on your journey, offering you additional "food for your soul"?*

# the "recipes" for success

Before you started reading this book, you may have flipped to the back to find the meal plan you are supposed to follow, or the recipes you should try. After all, these are a part of every other weight-loss or diet book you've ever read, right? Well, there *is* a "meal plan" included here—it's called "nourishment for your soul." And there are "recipes" provided as well—they're called "therapeutic recipes for success." But they're radically different from any meal plans or recipes you've seen before. *You've tried stuffing and starving your body, now try feeding your soul.*

The "recipes" outlined in this chapter give specific techniques for you to implement as nourishment for your soul. These are therapeutic techniques that I used on my own journey of freedom, and which I use in my workshops and counseling sessions with clients. There are thirty recipes, which are organized in a sequence that I recommend to facilitate learning the process of Intuitive Self-Care. When you try a recipe, take notes about your experience in your journal. Hold on to what you learned, and incorporate these new concepts into your everyday life. Let each recipe you try build on the previous ones. And don't just do them once—try each one again, record your new experiences in your journal, and then go back and reread your previous entries and observe your progress.

For those of you who want structure, follow one recipe a day for the next thirty days, in the order they are provided. For those who want more spontaneity, open randomly to a page in this chapter and follow whichever recipe you happen to turn to. For those of you ready to be intuitive, look within yourself and determine which principle you'd like to work on, then choose the recipe that seems the best for you in that moment. *"Feed" your soul in the way that works the best for you.*

Each recipe can serve one, two, ten, or more at a time. In other words, you can try these on your own, with a friend or therapist, or in a group setting. I've included the "ingredients" you'll need—materials like paper, crayons, scissors. I've also included an approximation of the time required to complete the outlined exercise. Of course, you can spend more or less time as needed. Note that each "recipe title" is an affirmation, which is a present-tense, positive statement that reflects what the recipe will cover in more detail.

I've always enjoyed cooking, but even if you don't, these recipes are easy and fun to try. Go ahead. Have some fun! *Nourishing your soul involves enjoying the process of your journey of freedom.*

## HAPPINESS RECIPES

These six recipes are based on the principle of loving your Self, and are designed to help you find more happiness in your life experience. The recipes address the three aspects of loving your

Self: Feel good outside your body, feel good about your body, feel good in your body.

## Recipe #1: Feel Good Outside Your Body

This recipe involves loving who you are "outside of," or independent of, your body. In other words, this recipe helps you honor and value your unique personality, interests, and accomplishments. The goal here is to see yourself as more than merely a body, to appreciate all the wonderful things that you contribute to the world. However, if you stop here, it can lead to a denial of your body. I see this in many overweight clients, who look beyond their bodies' size and focus on their other gifts, talents, and abilities. They avoid the mirror, or if they look in the mirror they are blind to their real bodies. This is better than self-criticism, but the idea is not to "pretend" that you don't have a body.

## Recipes #6, #11, #16: Feel Good About Your Body

Now it's time to make peace with that image in the mirror, to see yourself accurately, as you really are, and yet be free of criticism. The key is to notice the size and shape of your body without judging it. It is also important to focus on the functions of your body rather than its size and shape. Many clients have incredibly distorted perceptions of their bodies—some clients see themselves as much fatter than they really are, others see themselves as thinner. The key is to see the reality, without judgment. To see your body through your soul's eyes, not your body's eyes. With your body's eyes, looks are deceiving. Through your soul's eyes, you see reality. Your body is the home for your soul. How does your soul see this body? Why is this body the shape and size that it is? How do your body and mind together serve your soul?

## Recipes #21, #26: Feel Good in Your Body

What's it like to be IN your body? When you think about feeling good about your body and all that you do in the world, it's from an "outside" perspective. But what about your soul's perspective from within? What does your soul experience as it feels your body's movements, thinks your mind's thoughts, and goes through your day-to-day life in the world? Although your soul doesn't judge your body, it wants the body that can best serve, help, and heal. Your soul wants your help to share its message with the world. Your soul knows that this is the body you have right now, and it will guide you in using your body in the most effective way. Your soul will also help you make any necessary changes to enhance your body's ability to fulfill your soul's purpose.

## HEALTH RECIPES

These six recipes are based on the principle of being true to your Self, and are designed to help you enjoy more health in your life experience. The recipes address the three aspects of being true to your Self: Eat with inner wisdom, exercise with inner wisdom, live with inner wisdom.

## Recipes #2, #7: Eat with Inner Wisdom

These recipes are designed to help you move beyond the "diet men-tality" and its rules of what you should and shouldn't eat. Your soul is guiding the way in making your food choices, including the type and amount of food, as well as when you need to eat. Your body needs to heal from the abuses of the ups-and-downs of weight gain and loss, from the periods of fasting and overstuffing. You have denied your body food that it needs, and you have forced your body to eat food that it didn't need. Pay more attention to your body's messages, and let your soul guide you in responding to your body's true needs.

## Recipes #12, #17: Exercise with Inner Wisdom

Beyond the rigid rules of grueling exercise regimens is the intuitive wisdom of your soul, offering you an ideal fitness plan tailored to your specific needs. What a great personal trainer you already have, right there, within you! These recipes guide you in determining the type and amount of exercise that is right for you, and in enjoying the fitness activities that you choose.

## Recipes #22, #27: Live with Inner Wisdom

Eating and exercise choices are important for a healthy body, but what about a healthy mind and a healthy life? Your soul's wisdom is also guiding you in making healthy choices in all areas of your life.

## BALANCE RECIPES

These six recipes are based on the principle of expressing your Self, and are designed to help you enjoy more balance in your emotional life experience. The recipes address the three aspects of expressing your Self: Express your present concerns, express your past issues, express your core essence.

## Recipes #3, #8, #13: Express Your Present Concerns

To uncover some of those dark emotions, it's helpful to begin with the issues that you are presently grappling with. Certain thoughts and feelings will be most obvious to you, the foreground of a picture. Although these are your "present" concerns, they are usually regrets from the past or worries about the future that you are emphasizing at the present moment. Bringing these concerns to your conscious awareness is the first step in being able to experience your emotions, hear and learn their messages, and be in balance.

## Recipe #18: Express Your Past Issues

As you allow your emotions to surface, you will begin to discern recognizable patterns. Present issues often occur in the same or similar forms as in the past; these patterns can help us resolve past issues. They point the way to the deeper healing that we need to experience. You may notice that some old wounds seem to keep calling for your attention. You may find that those old wounds are triggering you to worry about future events. These old wounds are the unexpressed emotions from past issues that are calling for res- olution. This is the process of being the "emotional alchemist" who prepares dark emotions to be converted into a usable form.

## Recipes #23, #28: Express Your Core Essence

These recipes complete the process of "emotional alchemy," revealing the light amidst the darkness and transmuting the dark- ness into light. Your soul will reveal its wisdom and will guide you in this process. Here, you learn to appreciate the presence of all your emotions, experiencing a sense of happiness amidst sorrow, peace amidst chaos, and confidence amidst uncertainty. You learn to "feel with your soul," and you find your own balance amidst the ebb and flow of emotions.

## PEACE RECIPES

These six recipes are based on the principle of giving to your Self, and are designed to help you enjoy more peace in your life experience. The recipes address the three aspects of giving to your Self: Start the flow, enhance the flow, share the flow.

## Recipes #4, #9: Start the Flow

These recipes allow you to get the flow of peace going. This involves evaluating your current priorities and making changes as necessary to be able to meet more of your own needs. Just as you would have to find the space to dig a well, you need to clear a space in your own life where you can go "down and in" to tap into your soul. Starting the flow is about making the commitment to your Self.

## Recipes #14, #19: Enhance the Flow

Tapping the well to start the flow is just the beginning. Keeping the flow of peace going is the essential step. Many people tap into their soul for periods of time, then forget to attend to the flow, and the well dries up. Similarly, a real well will not continue to produce water on an ongoing basis if the well is not properly attended to. So, once you have started the flow going, once you have started to give to your Self, the key is to enhance the flow, to keep giving to your Self on a regular basis. These recipes involve establishing regular routines of Intuitive Self-Care.

## Recipes #24, #29: Share the Flow

Once your own peaceful flow is abundant, then you can give peace to others. Your flow will naturally lead you in the directions where you can best serve, help and heal. You can think of this as fulfilling your "life mission." Each of us has one. For some, it may involve a specific vocational "calling." For others, it's just a spiritual consciousness embraced during day-to-day life, with no specific vocation necessary. Only your soul knows how and where you can best give to others. You are being guided there. Trust the process.

## CONFIDENCE RECIPES

These six recipes are based on the principle of believing in your Self, and are designed to help you enjoy more confidence in your life experience. The recipes address the three aspects of believing in your Self: Celebrate past success, center current success, create ongoing success.

## Recipe #5: Celebrate Past Success

It's important to acknowledge every step that you take on your journey of freedom. Success builds on itself. Sometimes it may feel like you are on a lonely journey, and you may wonder if you are making any progress at all. It may even feel at times like you are regressing, losing ground. That's when it can be helpful to review all the progress that you have been making, and still are making.

## Recipes #10, #15, #20: Center Current Success

The "voices of the world" can have a powerful allure. While you may wish you could retreat entirely from the world, you will actually grow stronger by learning to "be in the world but not of the world"—staying as your true Self, a soul/mind/body in your everyday life. You may find yourself getting caught up in the world's demands, but you can always align your conscious awareness with the intuitive voice of your soul. These strategies help you remember that in this moment, you are already successful.

## Recipes #25, #30: Create Ongoing Success

Once you remember what you already know, having reconnected with your intuition, the key is to keep nourishing your soul to enhance the benefits you are now experiencing. With ongoing practice of everything that you have learned on your journey of freedom, you open the door to success in all areas of your life.

## Recipe #1 (Happiness): "I have greatness within me."

Ingredients: lined paper, pen or pencil, envelope with postage

Time required: 30 minutes

Directions: Your core beliefs and values say a great deal about who you really are. When you are clear about the beliefs and values that are truly important to you, then you can begin to live your life as a reflection of those values. Take out your piece of paper and write a letter, describing what your soul truly believes and values. Write this letter as if you'll be sending it to someone who doesn't know you. You might use headings like "I believe ..." and "I value ..." and then state why you feel that way. You might consider addressing topics such as a Higher Power, the meaning of life, and what happens when we die. Be creative. Let your soul really express itself. Once you have finished your letter, go back to the top of the page and write "Dear ___," filling your own name in the blank. At the end of your letter, write "Thanks for letting me experience this through you. I Love You, signed, your soul." After finishing the letter, say the affirmation: "I have greatness within me." Then put the letter in the envelope and mail it to yourself. When the letter arrives in the mail, open it and read it as if you are being given the information for the very first time. Read it with a sense of wonder, joy, and excitement. Read it with a sense of love, feeling the love your soul has for you.

Think about how you came to develop your beliefs and values. Who or what influenced your choices? Consider what you do when you meet someone whose values are different from yours. Do you stand up and defend your values? Are there some that you might abandon? How important are these beliefs and values to you? After reflecting, repeat the affirmation: "I have greatness within me."

## Recipe #2 (Health): "I am in tune with my body's hunger."

Ingredients: your body, several index cards

Time required: 2 minutes (repeat any time you feel hungry)

Directions: When you notice the sensation of hunger in your body, take time to "check in" with this feeling more deeply. Begin by noting the date and time on one side of an index card. Now, notice what your hunger feels like. Is it an ebbing, a gnawing, an emptiness, a tingling, a growling? Where do you notice it in your body? Is it in your stomach, your head, your entire body? How intense is the hunger? Are you a little hungry or do you feel starved? On a scale of 1 to 10, where 1 is empty/intense hunger and 10 is full/no hunger, how would you rank your hunger level? Record all of this information on the front side of your index card. Next, check in with the type and amount of food that you are hungry for. Note the general taste, texture, temperature. Do you want something sweet or sour, crunchy or chewy, hot or cold? Note the type of food you'd like. Describe it as the food itself, or as its constituents of protein, carbohydrate, fat, or a combination thereof. What would you like the food to do in your body, give you a quick burst of energy or be a lasting source of fuel? How much food do you think is required to satisfy your need? Record the specifics about the type and amount of food your body needs on the back side of the index card. Can you provide this food for your body to satisfy your true hunger? If not, what is a close substitute that you can make? Write any additional comments that you would like about this "check-in" experience. As you conclude this activity, say "I am in tune with my body's hunger."

Which questions were the easiest to answer? The hardest? What new information did you learn about your body and your hunger? As you repeat this activity, how can you use the information that you gather? After reflecting, repeat the affirmation: "I am in tune with my body's hunger."

## Recipe #3 (Balance):"I find resolution for my present concerns."

---

Ingredients: lined paper, pen or pencil

Time required: 15 minutes

Directions: Our minds tend to be filled with constant chatter, unconsciously hashing over all of our past regrets and future worries. Bringing these concerns to your present conscious awareness allows you to deal with them appropriately. On your sheet of paper, list anything that seems to be cluttering your mind right now. Write down any thoughts about what you have to do in the future, or concerns about what you didn't do in the past. Note any feelings that you have toward any person or situation. Review your list. Place an asterisk by any items that really stand out for you, anything that you feel requires your immediate attention. Pick one item with an asterisk, and write this concern at the top of the back side of your paper. What steps can you take to address the situation? If there is no action that you can take on this situation at the present time, then what steps can you take to accept it, exactly as it is? Repeat this process for the remainder of the items by which you placed an asterisk. As you complete this activity, say the affirmation: "I find resolution for my present concerns."

—◆—

*What was this experience like? How did it feel to bring all of the chatter in your mind to your conscious awareness? What kinds of action steps did you come up with, to either address or accept your concerns? After reflecting, repeat the affirmation: "I find resolution for my present concerns."*

## Recipe #4 (Peace): "I am open and receptive to give to my Self."

**Ingredients:** lined paper, pen or pencil

**Time required:** 10 minutes

**Directions:** You may be living a very busy and demanding life, and you may find it difficult to imagine how you can find the time to give to your Self. Take a few minutes to examine the ways in which you are spending your time. Are there some things that you can eliminate or at least cut back on so that you have more time to honor your own needs? Make a list of all the different people, events, commitments, and other activities that currently require your attention. Place an asterisk next to the activities that you really enjoy, which energize you, which seem to give back as much to you as you give to them. Place an X by the activities that you resist, which drain you, which seem to take more from you than you get back. Now, scan your list. How many asterisks do you have? How many X's? How many items have neither? Which X's can you eliminate? If you can't eliminate them, how can you convert them to an asterisk, or to being at least neutral? How can you convert some of your neutrals to asterisks? Are there some activities that you don't currently engage in but would like to add to your list, with asterisks? Write these down. As you conclude this activity, say the affirmation: "I am open and receptive to give to my Self."

——

*What did you learn as you made your list? How can you make changes to your list so that your time is filled with activities that meet your needs and the needs of others? After reflecting, repeat the affirmation: "I am open and receptive to give to my Self."*

## Recipe #5 (Confidence): "I am confident and successful."

**Ingredients:** lined paper or journal, pen or pencil

**Time required:** 10 minutes

**Directions:** Expressing gratitude for what is working in your life is a powerful way to attract more success. Being grateful for what you'd like to experience in your life before it happens is even more powerful. On your paper or in your journal, write down the various things that you are grateful for that have already happened. For example, "I am thankful for being more in tune with my body's hunger and fullness levels," or "I appreciate the enhanced connection I have with the voice of my soul." Next, list your gratitude for what is in the process of unfolding in your life. For example, "I am thankful for being at the Freedom point," or, "I am grateful for my ongoing success." As you conclude this activity, say "I am confident and successful."

———

*What was this experience like? What would happen if you made time to express your gratitude on a daily basis? After reflecting, repeat the affirmation: "I am confident and successful."*

## Recipe #6 (Happiness): "I am free of the ideals of the world."

Ingredients: two fashion/fitness magazines

Time required: 15 minutes

Description: We tend to be inundated with messages from the world, telling us how we should look, act, think, and live our lives. It is only when we compare our Self with the world's standards that we begin to think, "I'm not good enough." A key to Self-love is letting go of the world's ideals. Flip through a fashion or fitness magazine, and each time you see an image or words that convey an "ideal" standard, rip the page out. After you have gone through the entire magazine, how many pages are left? Now, taking the pages you have ripped out, review each one and try to look past the ideal that's being presented. Just see it as a person or an object or words on a page, without assigning a judgment to it, either positive or negative. What would happen if you could do that for all advertisements? Now, take another magazine and flip through it, remaining neutral to its messages, observing but not being controlled by the messages. After you finish flipping through the second magazine, say to yourself: "I am free of the ideals of the world."

———

*What was your overall experience like? How did it feel to rip the pages out? Then to go back through them free of judgment? After completing this activity for the first time, do you really feel free of the ideals of the world? It may take a few repetitions of this activity for you to feel completely free. What else would help you to stay neutral to the world's ideals? After reflecting, repeat the affirmation: "I am free of the ideals of the world."*

## Recipe #7 (Health): "I offer my body a variety of food choices."

Ingredients: plain paper, pen or pencil

Time required: 15 minutes

Directions: Turn your sheet of paper lengthwise, and draw four columns. Label the columns "Breakfast," "Lunch," "Dinner," and "Snacks." Under each heading, write some ideas of different foods that you could offer your body. Make your menu selections from foods that you have in your kitchen or that you can readily purchase. Also consider ease of preparation. Let go of any "diet rules," and consider the foods that will best nourish your body. List complete meal choices with some flexibility, such as "Hot or cold cereal with soy milk and fresh fruit," or "Grilled fish with wild rice or potatoes, and a green vegetable." Try to list at least three menu choices in each category. When your menu is finished, review your list and say the affirmation: "I offer my body a variety of food choices." Post your completed menu on your refrigerator or a cupboard in your kitchen. Then, the next time you are hungry but feel unable to determine what you are hungry for, scan your menu. As you read the descriptions of each item, pay attention to how that selection would satisfy your hunger at the moment, and make the choice that is closest to your current need. Keep in mind that sometimes you may want a breakfast item for dinner, or vice versa. Each time you make a food choice from your menu, repeat the affirmation: "I offer my body a variety of food choices."

—◆—

*What was important to you in choosing your menu items? Did you list only foods that are familiar, or did you also include some new possibilities? Why or why not? How will having this menu help you with responding to your hunger? When do you plan to update your menu? After reflecting, repeat the affirmation: "I offer my body a variety of food choices."*

## Recipe #8 (Balance): "I recognize the messages my symptoms are sending me."

---

**Ingredients:** plain paper, pen or pencil

**Time required:** 30 minutes

**Directions:** Your eating, exercise, and other weight-related symptoms are trying to tell you something. But what? Look more closely at your various symptoms, and discover their messages. Turn your paper lengthwise, and make four columns. Label the columns "Symptom," "Purpose," "True Need," and "How to Meet this Need" In the first column, list the various eating, exercise, and weight symptoms that you experience. For example, "Binge eating, overeating sugary foods, feeling fat, skipping meals." The "purpose" of each listed symptom is the perceived need you are trying to get it to fill. For binge eating, you may list the purpose as, "To stuff down, numb or escape from feelings." Next, what is the true need (rather than the purpose)? The symptom is an attempt to meet the perceived need, but what is the true need? In the case of binge eating, you might say "To feel comforted and secure during times of difficult emotions." Finally, list at least one alternative way that you can meet your need, instead of using the symptom. For example, rather than binge eating, you could call a friend for comfort. As you complete this activity, say the affirmation: "I recognize the messages my symptoms are sending me."

---

*What patterns did you discover in your responses? How often do you currently use your symptoms instead of meeting your true needs? What would help you to meet your true needs more often? After reflecting, repeat the affirmation: "I recognize the messages my symptoms are sending me."*

## Recipe #9 (Peace): "I give my Self what I truly need."

**Ingredients:** lined paper, pen or pencil

**Time required:** 15 minutes

**Directions:** How are you re-parenting yourself? Consider what you are "feeding" yourself—what you are giving to your body, mind, and soul. Do you have some needs that remain unmet? At the top of one sheet of paper, write "What my soul wants for my body." Then list some soulful things you'd like to "feed" your body. Think about the food choices you are making, and any changes your soul is calling for you to make. Consider your exercise choices as well. How can you give your body what it really needs? On a second sheet of paper, write "What my soul wants for my mind." Make a list of some things you'd like to "feed" your mind. What kinds of academic pursuits would you enjoy? How else is your soul guiding you to nourish your mind? On a third sheet of paper, write "What my soul wants for itself." What are you doing to "feed" your soul, and how can you enhance this list? What types of spiritual practice would be meaningful to you? As you conclude this activity, say "I give my Self what I truly need."

———

*Have you been overfeeding—or underfeeding—yourself? Which is the most "hungry"—your body, mind, or soul? What's it like to be on the receiving end? Do you like what you are giving to your Self? On the other hand, what's it like to be on the giving end? How does it feel to give to your Self? After reflecting, repeat the affirmation: "I give my Self what I truly need."*

## Recipe #10 (Confidence): "In this moment, I believe in my Self."

Ingredients: plain paper, pen or pencil

Time required: 15 minutes

Directions: Turn your paper lengthwise, and draw three vertical lines to make three columns. In the left column, write "Regrets." List all of the concerns that you have about "mistakes" you made a few minutes ago, yesterday, last week, or any time in the past. In the right column, write "Worries." List all of the concerns that you have about "mistakes" you could make in a few minutes, tomorrow, next week, or any time in the he future. Look over each of these two columns. How do you feel? Now fold your paper in thirds, tucking the "Regrets" and "Worries" behind so that only the center section is available for you to see. In the center of this column, write the word "NOW" in capital letters. In this moment, *right now,* what concerns do you have? Are you aware of any, *right now?* Where would you rather put your focus—in the past, the future, or the present moment? As you conclude this activity, say "In this moment, I believe in my Self."

— —

*What was this experience like? Did you list anything in your center column? What would you like to fill your NOW with? After reflecting, repeat the affirmation: "In this moment, I believe in my Self."*

## Recipe #11 (Happiness): "I accept my Self, exactly as I am."

**Ingredients:** lined paper, pen or pencil

**Time required:** 20 minutes

**Directions:** Draw a line down the middle of a sheet of paper, to make two columns. In the left column, write any critical or negative thoughts that you have about who you are or how you look. These might include "I'm a failure," "I'm not good enough," "I'm a fat pig," or "My thighs look like tree trunks." Get all the negative thoughts out of your head and onto your paper. Then, scan your list. How do you feel? Now imagine that your best friend has just rattled off all those criticisms about herself. How would you reply? Reread each criticism, and then in the right column write your "response to my friend." Develop a new, positive statement, not merely a rebuttal of the old negative one. For example, don't write "You are not a failure." Highlight the positive, such as "You have succeeded at many things—for example, you were recently promoted at work and your photography won an award." In response to "I'm not good enough," you might respond "You have many wonderful qualities, including a great sense of humor and a giving nature." To "I'm a fat pig," you could say "You have beautiful eyes." For the tree-trunk-thighs example, focus on the function of legs while de-emphasizing their size, responding "Your strong thighs allow you to walk, stand, and climb." If you get stuck framing a positive message, ask someone to help you. After you've completed your list, scan both columns. How do you feel? Now, fold your paper in half. Read only the right side. How do you feel? As you conclude the activity, say the affirmation: "I accept my Self, exactly as I am."

*What was your overall experience while doing this activity? Do you believe the positive statements you wrote in the right column? Can you accept your Self, even if you still perceive that you have flaws? How can you be more accepting? After reflecting, repeat the affirmation: "I accept my Self, exactly as I am."*

## Recipe #12 (Health): "I am soulful as I eat."

Ingredients: your body, several index cards

Time required: 2 minutes (repeat any time you eat)

Directions: When you are eating, "check in" with your body and think about how the meal is satisfying you. Take an index card and note the date and the time that you are beginning to enjoy your meal. Now let your eating be a soulful experience. Really tune in and pay attention to what eating feels like. How does the food feel in your mouth? Notice the temperature, texture, and taste of the food. Is this what you wanted? Is it satisfying you? What do you like about it? As you swallow, notice how the food feels while traveling to your stomach, and how it feels once it is in your stomach. Notice how your stomach feels as you eat more. What other changes do you notice in your body? Do you feel energized? Calm? Anxious? Where do you notice these feelings in your body? Record all of this information on the front side of your index card. As you start to get full, turn your index card over to record some additional information. First, record the time, and notice how much time has passed since you started eating. Tune in to what the early signs of fullness feel like. Describe them, and where you feel them in your body. How full do you feel? Describe it in words: "Satisfied," "Full," or perhaps "Stuffed." Next, rate your fullness on a scale of 1 to 10, where 1 is empty/intense hunger and 10 is full/no hunger. Do you choose to continue eating, or have you had enough? If you continue, notice what it feels like as you eat more. When you finish eating, make any additional comments that you would like about your eating experience. As you conclude this activity, say the affirmation: "I am soulful as I eat."

*Which questions were the easiest to answer? The hardest? What new information did you learn about your body and your fullness? As you repeat this activity, how can you use the information that you gather? After reflecting, repeat the affirmation: "I am soulful as I eat."*

## Recipe #13 (Balance): "I express my emotions in healthy ways."

Ingredients: lined paper, pen or pencil, art materials, music

Time required: 30 minutes

Directions: Remember being a little kid, when you got to write stories, draw pictures, and dance to music? You were actually doing something very healthy for yourself, because each of those activities was a form of emotional expression. Those same things can be helpful for you right now, today. Begin by tuning in to the feeling that is strongest right now. Do you feel happy? Afraid? Depressed? Excited? Worried? Once you have labeled your feeling, spend a few minutes writing about what that feeling means. Don't worry about grammar or spelling, just let your insights flow freely onto the page. After a few minutes, go on to your art materials. Use crayons, colored pencils, finger paints, or any other materials that you choose, and capture the essence of your feeling visually. Don't worry about the quality of your artwork: It's fine to simply splash colors and shapes onto the page. After spending some time trying art, move on to music. Select a type of music that fits your mood, and either listen to it or play a musical instrument. If you listen to the music, try moving your body in a way that captures the essence of how you feel. After you have tried all three modes of expression—the written word, visual art, music—return to the one that was most effective for you, and complete the expression of your emotion. After completing this activity, say the affirmation: "I express my emotions in healthy ways."

Which of the three modes of expression worked best for you: writing, art, or music? Why? Are there certain emotions that you think you'd choose to express with different modes? Can you think of other healthy ways to express how you feel? After reflecting, repeat the affirmation: "I express my emotions in healthy ways."

## Recipe #14 (Peace): "I receive the gifts I already have."

Ingredients: a box with a lid, wrapping paper, scissors, tape, paper, pen or pencil

Time required: 20 minutes

Directions: Sometimes it can feel like you only give, but never receive. Now you can enjoy a gift any time you need one—a gift from your Self. Using the wrapping paper, wrap the lid of your box and then cover the body of the box as well. Next, cut the paper into medium-sized pieces. On each piece, write something that you are currently doing to meet your needs. For example, "I go to bed by 10:00 P.M. and enjoy a restful sleep," or "I feed my body the food that I am really hungry for." Then, deposit all the nurturing notes into the box. Put the lid on your box, and then hold it as you say "I give this gift to my Self." Now, open the box and read all the nurturing notes out loud. After you have read each one, put the notes back inside. As you complete this activity, say "I receive the gifts I already have."

*What was it like to do this activity? How was it to receive a gift from your Self? How can you use this gift in the future? How can you enhance your gift? After reflecting, repeat the affirmation: "I receive the gifts I already have."*

## Recipe #15 (Confidence): "I easily move beyond any obstacles on my path."

Ingredients: lined paper, pen or pencil

Time required: 10 minutes

Directions: As you continue on your journey of freedom, you may notice some challenges. These obstacles can be opportunities for you to succeed! On your paper, make two columns. In the left column, write the heading "Obstacles." List anything that seems to be difficult for you right now. List it as a comment or a question. For example, "I still don't like my fat body," or "How can I cut back on my emotional eating?" In the right column, write the heading "Solutions." Read each comment or question, and then write a response from your soul. Go deep within yourself to write your reply in a gentle, loving, encouraging way. For example, in response to the comment about the "fat body," your soul might say "Your body is the size and shape it needs to be right now. Thank you for letting me experience you exactly the way you are." Regarding emotional eating, your soul might reply "What are you really 'hungry' for? Honor what you really need." If you have difficulty with any of your responses, imagine what you might say to a friend who had those same complaints or questions. As you conclude this activity, say "I easily move beyond any obstacles on my path."

---

*What was it like to write responses to yourself from your soul? What helped you to hear your soul's voice more easily? How can you use your soul's wisdom to help you succeed? After reflecting, repeat the affirmation: "I easily move beyond any obstacles on my path."*

## Recipe #16 (Happiness): "I see my whole Self with my soul's eyes."

**Ingredients**: a full-length and a hand-held mirror, post-it notes, pen or pencil

**Time required**: 10 minutes

**Directions**: Stand in front of a full-length mirror, fully clothed, and just look at your body. (A full-length mirror is best, but substitute a smaller-size mirror if necessary.) Regard yourself from the front, sides, and back (using the hand-held mirror). Look your body over, from head to toe. What do you see? Now, repeat this entire process using your soul's eyes of love. See your body only through eyes of love. Every time you see something positive, write it down on a post-it note. For example, "I like my hair" or "I have a nice smile." Look long enough to record at least five qualities. Now, look within yourself and see the positive aspects of your mind. Look within using your soul's eyes. As you notice something positive, write it on a post-it note. For example, "I am smart" or "I have a good sense of humor." Search long enough to record at least three qualities. Now, look even deeper within, to see your soul reflected back to you. What do you see? What positive aspects of your core essence are being revealed to you? Look long enough to get at least one quality. Write it down. As you conclude this activity, look at your whole Self in the mirror and say "I see my whole Self with my soul's eyes." Then, as a follow-up, take all your post-it notes and put them in various places where you'll notice them throughout your day: on mirrors, on the refrigerator door, on your car's dashboard, in your wallet.

—◆—

*What was this entire experience like for you? What parts of the activity were hardest? Easiest? What would happen if you repeated this activity again, but this time with an unclothed body? After reflecting, repeat the affirmation: "I see my whole Self with my soul's eyes."*

## Recipe #17 (Health): "I offer my body a variety of fitness choices."

---

Ingredients: plain paper, pen or pencil

Time required: 15 minutes

Directions: Turn your sheet of paper lengthwise, and divide it into three columns. Label the columns "Cardiovascular," "Strength," and "Flexibility." Under each heading, write a description of what each type of exercise means to you. For example, "Cardiovascular: moving quickly, heart rate up." Also, list benefits that you perceive, such as, "Strength: increased energy, injury prevention." Next, write some ideas of different fitness activities that you could offer your body within each category. Make your list based on activities that you enjoy, or would like to try. Let go of any "exercise rules," and consider the activities that will best nourish your body. If an activity falls under more than one category, enter it in all applicable columns. For example, yoga is good for both strength and flexibility, and many aerobics classes target both cardiovascular benefits and strength. Try to list at least three fitness choices in each category. When your list is finished, review it and say the affirmation: "I offer my body a variety of fitness choices." Post your completed list where you will see it at the time you designate for activity. Then, when that time comes but you feel unable to determine what type of activity you need, read your list. Pay attention to how that fitness choice would satisfy your body's need to move, and make the choice that is closest to your need. Each time you make a fitness choice using your list, repeat the affirmation: "I offer my body a variety of fitness choices."

As you made your list, what factors did you consider? How will having this list help you respond to your fitness needs? When do you plan to update your list? After reflecting, repeat the affirmation: "I offer my body a variety of fitness choices."

## Recipe #18 (Balance): "I release my attachment to my old wounds."

**Ingredients:** lined paper, pen or pencil

**Time required:** 30 minutes

**Directions:** Past traumas and old wounds can sometimes have a hidden appeal. Until you are willing to let go of your past issues, you will carry them with you like battle scars, often building your identity around these wounds. However, this can lock you into the role of "victim." Although you can't change your past, you can change your experience of the past in the present. You can free yourself of the need to carry the baggage of past issues. On your sheet of paper, make three columns. Label the columns "Old Wound," "Help," and "Harm." List any previous traumas or past issues that you have been holding onto. How has staying attached to each wound been helpful to you? What benefits are you getting by continuing to identify yourself with each wound? For example, if your old wound is the death of your mother when you were a small child, you may realize that holding onto this wound has allowed you to receive sympathy and attention from others. Now, consider how this identification has been holding you back. What harm does it cause you to hold onto each wound? For example, you may discover that you have been overeating to "replace the love you lost" upon your mother's death. Next, ask yourself if there is another way that you can get the benefits you listed in the "Help" column, instead of through that old wound. For example, you could receive attention for positive elements of your personality. In conclusion, acknowledge the purpose that your wound has been serving, and gently ask for it to be released, knowing that your needs can be met in other ways. As you complete this activity, say "I release my attachment to my old wounds."

— —

*What was this experience like? What has been your purpose in holding onto your old wounds? What is it like to know that you can meet your needs in other ways? After reflecting, repeat the affirmation: "I release my attachment to my old wounds."*

## Recipe #19 (Peace): "I follow a soulful routine."

**Ingredients:** lined paper, pen or pencil

**Time required:** 10 minutes

**Directions:** What is the purpose of a routine? To have something familiar. What is the purpose of a soulful routine? To have something soulfully familiar. Do you see the difference? Think about the different routines in your life. Your morning routine. Your workday routine. Your bedtime routine. Your family routine. What would it be like to include soulful practice in your everyday routines? First, think of some different things that you could do as part of your soulful practice. On the front side of your paper, make a list of your ideas: Meditation. Reading spiritual literature. Watching the sunrise. Prayer. Expressing gratitude at the end of the day. List anything that you feel would nourish your soul and enhance your conscious awareness of your core essence. Next, think about when you can incorporate these activities into your daily life. Perhaps you can make some of them part of your morning routine, and others part of your bedtime routine. Some activities you can do in solitude, but you may choose to do others with other people. Try to incorporate one or two of your ideas at a time. Note your plans on your paper. As you conclude this activity, say "I follow a soulful routine."

*What kinds of routines do you currently follow? How do you plan to incorporate soulful activities into your daily routines? What do you think will be different with more soulful activities as part of your lifestyle? After reflecting, repeat the affirmation: "I follow a soulful routine."*

## Recipe #20 (Confidence): "I am centered in my soul."

**Ingredients:** a quiet space, your body, an index card, pen or pencil

**Time required:** 15 minutes

**Directions:** Sit comfortably in your quiet space, and close your eyes. Take several deep breaths, and relax. Feel the connection with your soul. Experience the confidence of being a soul/mind/body. Take several deep breaths and feel the energy within you, moving through you with a sense of confidence. Now, let your thoughts drift back out to the world. What concerns do you perceive? What challenges do you anticipate? What problems do you imagine? Notice how this feels in your body as you let your mind pay attention to the world. Now, let the world go. Bring your mind back to your soul. What can you tell your mind to help you with this process of reconnection? Say a simple word or phrase to assist you: for example, "Center," or "I am connected." Repeat this word or phrase to yourself. Notice how you feel in your body. Take several deep breaths and feel the energy within you, moving through you with a sense of confidence. Sit in this space of confidence as long as you wish. When you conclude this time of meditation, write the word or phrase that you used on your index card. As you conclude this activity, say "I am centered in my soul."

*What was your word or phrase? How can you use your index card as a reminder to help you stay centered in your soul? After reflecting, repeat the affirmation: "I am centered in my soul."*

## Recipe #21 (Happiness): "I enjoy being in my body."

**Ingredients:** your body, a place to walk

**Time required:** 10 minutes

**Directions:** Go to a place where you will have some room to move, preferably outdoors. While standing still, close your eyes and take a few deep breaths. Notice how it feels to simply breathe. Feel the air filling your lungs as you inhale, and feel your body move as you exhale. Raise your arms overhead, and stand on your tip-toes, stretching up as tall as you can get. Feel the whole length of your body. Lower your arms, and extend them straight in front of you. Swing your arms from side to side, your arms stretched out, and feel the breadth of your body. Stand still again, breathing. Inhale deeply, noticing any scents around you. Use your ears and listen to all the sounds around you. Open your eyes. Take in the view around you. Now, take a few steps in any direction. Notice how it feels to be in your body. As you walk, feel the movement of every part of your body: hands, arms, feet, legs, buttocks, back, head. Feel the air on your skin. Stop and touch something, perhaps a leaf or some blades of grass. Notice its texture and temperature. Continue to walk, slowly at first, and then speeding up. Notice the difference in how you feel in your body as you move at different speeds. As you conclude this activity, think about how grateful you are for the body you have, and say "I enjoy being in my body."

---

*What did you notice as you did this activity? When did you feel most comfortable in your body? When were you least comfortable? After reflecting, repeat the affirmation: "I enjoy being in my body."*

## Recipe #22 (Health): "I am soulful as I exercise."

Ingredients: your body, a place to move

Time required: 10 minutes

Directions: Stand with your feet spaced a comfortable distance apart. Take several deep breaths, and notice how it feels as the air fills and is released from your lungs. Repeat this breathing process several times, paying attention to your inner experience. How does your body feel? Your mind? Your soul? Now, march in place, moving your arms by your sides and lifting your knees to a moderate height. Take note of your inner experience. How does your body feel? Your mind? Your soul? Check in with your soul. What other movements do you want to experience? Moving side to side? Jumping as high as you can? Bending and twisting? Just breathing again? As you conclude this activity, say "I am soulful as I exercise."

———

*What was different about the experience for your body, mind, and soul? The next time you exercise, tune in to your inner experience. What do you think will be different? After reflecting, repeat the affirmation: "I am soulful as I exercise."*

## Recipe #23 (Balance): "I find the light amidst the darkness."

**Ingredients:** lined paper, pen or pencil

**Time required:** 30 minutes

**Directions:** There is a saying, "The tallest trees have weathered many storms." Through the "storms" in your life, you can grow stronger. Another adage is "Every cloud has a silver lining." Every difficult experience has within it the potential for a positive experience. Your struggles can be opportunities for growth, if you choose to find the light amidst the darkness. Let one of your current problems come to mind. Take a piece of paper and write some details about this problem. Describe the problem from the perspective of the "chatter" in your mind. Now, go beyond the surface level of the problem, go deep within yourself, digging down to your soul. From your soul's perspective, what is this problem all about? What's the bigger picture? What are the emotions you find here to teach you? What positive experience can you take away from what seems like adversity? What strength can you gain? What silver lining can you find? How can this seeming problem be a blessing in disguise? Turn your paper over, and write about your problem from this new perspective of your soul. As you conclude this activity, say "I find the light amidst the darkness."

—◆—

*Which perspective do you prefer, that of the chatter in your mind or the wisdom of your soul? What did you learn about your problem? Are there other problems that you would like to repeat this process with? After reflecting, repeat the affirmation: "I find the light amidst the darkness."*

## Recipe #24 (Peace): "I am here to be truly helpful."

**Ingredients:** lined paper, pen or pencil

**Time required:** 20 minutes

**Directions:** You may feel that you have a purpose for being here, that there is some way you are to make a difference in the world. But what is it? You can gain clarity and an understanding of what your life purpose may be by expressing *how* you intend to live. In other words, define the values, beliefs, and standards that are the framework of your life. Just as companies have mission statements that define the principles they represent, you can write a mission statement for your own life. To begin this process, ask your soul "How may I be truly helpful?" Then take note of the insights you receive. Write out a few words or sentences that capture the essence of your personal mission statement. As you conclude this activity, say "I am here to be truly helpful."

— —

*What did you learn from this activity? How can you use your personal mission statement now that you have it? After reflecting, repeat the affirmation: "I am here to be truly helpful."*

## Recipe #25 (Confidence): "I believe in my Self and my ongoing success."

**Ingredients:** poster board, old magazines, scissors, glue stick

**Time required:** 45 minutes

**Directions:** A collage of words and pictures can be an excellent means by which to anchor your success, since visual reminders are very powerful. To make your own "success collage," begin by placing all of your materials on a large table or spread them on the floor. Spend 20 minutes flipping through the pages of your magazines, tearing out any pictures or words that represent your success. Work quickly, without analyzing the words or pictures. Go with an intuitive response to what you see. After 20 minutes, stop looking through the magazines. Spend the next 15 minutes preparing what you have collected, cutting out the right words from the pages, or tearing if you prefer. Spend the final 10 minutes arranging your pictures and words on your poster board. Don't think too hard about the placement, just go with your intuition. Use the glue stick to secure your items on the board. After concluding this activity, say "I believe in my Self and my ongoing success."

———

*What was this experience like? What are the key messages that you have included on your collage? How do you interpret the placement of your items? How can this collage help you with your ongoing success? After reflecting, repeat the affirmation: "I believe in my Self and my ongoing success."*

## Recipe #26 (Happiness): "I am seeing with my soul."

**Ingredients:** your body, an open space to stand

**Time required:** 10 minutes

**Directions:** Stand with your feet spaced a comfortable distance apart. Close your eyes, and take several deep breaths. As you inhale, raise your arms overhead and imagine that you are taking in happiness with every breath. As you exhale, lower your arms and imagine that you are extending happiness out into the world. Breathe in happiness, exhale happiness. Repeat this exercise several times. Then, focus attention on your feet. Let them feel firmly rooted, as if they extended down into the earth's core, like the roots of a giant tree. Now, imagine you are that tree. Extend your arms up and out, or keep them close to your sides, serving as your branches. Move your arms move back and forth, as if they were branches swaying in the wind. Let your body extend as tall as you can get, as if the tree were growing taller, reaching toward the sky. Now, be still, and simply enjoy the experience of being in your body, as the "tree of me." Continue to take happiness in as you inhale, and exhale happiness out into the world. Now, slowly open your eyes. What do you notice? How do your surroundings appear? As you conclude this activity, say "I am seeing with my soul."

———

*What was it like to be IN your body during this activity? What does the metaphor of being a tree mean to you? What are your "roots"? Your "branches"? Your "trunk"? How do these serve a purpose for you and others? How do you interact with the world? After reflecting, repeat the affirmation: "I am seeing with my soul."*

## Recipe #27 (Health): "I am thinking with my soul."

**Ingredients:** your body, a quiet space

**Time required:** 10 minutes

**Directions:** Sit comfortably in your quiet space, and close your eyes. Take several deep breaths to help you relax. Now, imagine that you are planting a garden. First, visualize the space where you will plant your garden. What does it look like? Is it ready for planting, or does the soil need to be prepared first? Once the ground is ready, imagine that you reach into your pocket and pull out three seeds. The first seed represents "eating with intuition," the second represents "exercise with intuition," and the third represents "life with intuition." Carefully put each seed into the ground. What do you need to help these seeds grow? Now, you notice the seeds have started to sprout. As the shoots emerge, what do they look like? Is there anything impeding their growth? What do you need to do to take care of your garden? As you complete the activity, say "I am thinking with my soul."

---

*What needed to be "cleared away" before you could plant your garden? Did you water your seeds, and what does the water represent? What else did you do to help your seeds grow? What was impeding their growth? What else did you discover? After reflecting, repeat the affirmation: "I am thinking with my soul."*

## Recipe #28 (Balance): "I am feeling with my soul."

**Ingredients:** your body, a quiet space

**Time required:** 10 minutes

**Directions:** Sometimes it helps to "turn over" a problem to the wisdom of your soul. Bring to your awareness any difficult situations, unresolved issues, or other emotional concerns. Choose one or several that you would like to release. Sit comfortably in your quiet space. Imagine that you are walking along a pathway, and you are carrying these problems with you. Are you carrying them in your body, on your body, or close to your body? Get a sense of what these problems look and feel like to you. Now, as you walk further down the pathway, you notice a bright light ahead of you. The light invites you to give your problems to it. Now, imagine that you let go of your problems. Get a sense of what that looks like, as the problems go from inside of you, on you, or around you, and move into the light. What happens to them as they touch the light? What wisdom is revealed to you as you release these problems into the light? Is there anything you want to ask or say to the light? As you conclude this activity, say the affirmation: "I am feeling with my soul."

---

*What was this experience like? What did you learn about your problems? What did you learn about and from the light? After reflecting, repeat the affirmation: "I am feeling with my soul."*

## Recipe #29 (Peace): "I am acting with my soul."

**Ingredients:** your body, a quiet space

**Time required:** 10 minutes

**Directions:** Sit comfortably in your quiet space, with your eyes closed. Imagine that you are taking a walk out in the wilderness, when you notice a small trickle of water coming from the ground. You feel very peaceful as you observe the water flowing. The more peaceful you feel, the more the water flows. Your own peace seems to be what is feeding this natural spring. The flow increases now into a stream. Imagine that you step into the stream, to fully experience the flow. You can ride in a boat or float in the water. Just relax into the flow. Be in peace as the stream carries you where you are meant to go. Where is the flow taking you? Stay in peace as you let your soul guide you onward in this visualization. Stay in the flow as long as you choose. As you conclude this activity, say "I am acting with my soul."

*What kind of wilderness did you imagine? Where did the flow begin? Where did it take you? What does this mean to you about your own life purpose? After reflecting, repeat the affirmation: "I am acting with my soul."*

## Recipe #30 (Confidence): "I am being with my soul."

**Ingredients:** your body, a quiet space

**Time required:** 10 minutes

**Directions:** Sit comfortably in your quiet space. Take several deep breaths, and relax. As you inhale, breathe in freedom. As you exhale, release any tension, heaviness, or burdens that you may have been carrying with you. As you inhale, feel yourself getting lighter. As you exhale, imagine that heavy blankets are being lifted away. With each exhalation, you release more of the weight that has been burdening your soul. With each inhalation, you feel your soul becoming more free. As the last heavy blanket is lifted away, all that is left is a beautiful, colorful balloon. Notice its size and shape. Is it a small helium balloon? A giant hot air balloon? Notice all the details about this balloon you have uncovered. Now, become the balloon, and drift gently into the air. Feel how light and free you are! No more weight to hold you back! No more burdens to worry about! Enjoy the experience of complete and total freedom. In this moment, how much does your soul weigh? Stay in this experience as long as you choose. As you conclude this activity, say "I am being with my soul."

—◦—

*What was this experience like? What do the blankets represent? What does your balloon represent? How much does your soul weigh? What will help your soul to be light and free? After reflecting, repeat the affirmation: "I am being with my soul."*

# enjoy your journey
# of freedom

*How much does your soul weigh?*

Does your soul feel more light and free? What have you been doing—or *not* doing—that is helping your soul feel this way? You have probably let go of your dieter's bag of burdens. What is it like to be free of the diet mentality, and its apathetic and obsessive extremes? You have likely been practicing Intuitive Self-Care, the process that naturally thin people have known their entire lives. What is it like to ACT AS IF you've never had a weight problem? You have probably released the barriers that were in the way of your own intuition. What is it like to reconnect with your soul's wisdom? You have probably been nourishing your soul with "recipes" for success. How does it feel to be feeding your hungry soul?

*How much does your soul weigh?*

Have you noticed that the more you feed your soul, the lighter and freer it becomes? What is happening to your body, the more that you nourish your soul? How are your eating, exercise, and weight symptoms changing? Are you aware of any shifts in your body's shape and size? When you are living from the inside out as a soul/mind/body, what is your life experience like? When you see, think, feel, act, and be with your soul, what do you notice? What is it like to be your true Self, to be who you really are? Express gratitude with each step you take on your journey and remain patient with the process. Do you notice a shift in your happiness, health, balance, peace, and confidence? Take the Self-Test in Appendix I again, and compare your current results with the score you obtained when you first started reading this book. Celebrate the success you now enjoy, and know there is much more to come.

*How much does your soul weigh?*

Your soul may feel more light and free than it has ever been. This book has offered you the support to begin your journey. But what happens next? You are like a child who is learning to ride a bicycle—you've started out with training wheels and you've learned to cruise along pretty well. But now it's time to take the training wheels off the bike. You are ready to ride on your own. You are ready to go more deeply within yourself to access the wisdom of your soul to help you continue on your way. Think about what happens to that child when she tries her first ride without the training wheels. She may fall a few times, which can be painful and discouraging. Similarly, you may "fall" by reverting back to your old diet patterns or eating-disorder symptoms. Don't give up. The key is to keep believing that you can succeed, and to stay connected with your soul's wisdom. It may be helpful for you to reread this book several times. Each time you read it, be prepared to discover something new. Take notes in your journal.

Depending on where you are on your journey of life, different elements will resonate with you. Highlight the concepts in this book that seem to be your own soul speaking to you. Put these into practice, in the most soulful manner that you can. Record your progress and insights in your journal as you continue on your journey of freedom. Remember, your journal is an essential tool for your ongoing success!

*How much does your soul weigh?*

Your soul can be even lighter and freer than it is now. The child learning to ride a bicycle gets better with practice. So can you. Keep practicing the process of Intuitive Self-Care. How do you feel when you are really in tune with your soul? *Be present.* Remind yourself to see, think, feel, act, and be with your soul. From this sacred space of your core essence, you can enjoy a magnificent experience on your journey, now and in each moment. The child on her bicycle can prevent falls from happening. So can you. Catch yourself whenever you are drawn by the voices of the world, instead of honoring the voice of your soul. This indicates that you are straying from the path and heading for a "fall." How do you feel when this happens? *Be aware.* Pay attention to the subtle signs that indicate you are falling out of touch with your intuition. Make adjustments to get back on track. The child on her bicycle knows that if she falls, she can recover quickly. So can you. You may not catch the subtle signs that you are shifting from a soul/mind/body back to a world/mind/body. It may take a "fall" back into your old symptoms—from apathy to obsession, from anorexia to obesity. *Be conscious.* If old symptoms show up, make the choice to stay centered in your essence as you observe them and learn from them. Let your life be your teacher.

*How much does your soul weigh?*

Your soul can stay light and free, even if you "fall." Don't measure your success by the absence of your symptoms. *Measure success by the presence of your soul.* You are free as long as you are experiencing your life from the inside out, as a soul/mind/body. Even after mastering bicycle riding, there still may be times when that child will fall. An obstacle on the road may throw her, the bicycle may malfunction, or she may just lose her balance for no apparent reason. Similarly, months or years after you are free, after you think you know all there is to know about Intuitive Self-Care, you may "fall" again. For example, you may revert back to your old overeating patterns, and as a result, regain some of the weight you lost when you initially followed this program. If this happens, it does not mean you have failed! Honor what is. *The return of any symptoms is a call for more soul.* It's an opportunity to enhance your awareness of your soul, to take all that you have learned to an even deeper level, and to practice conscious choice. Strengthen your commitment to Intuitive Self-Care. Reread this book, and review the notes in your journal. Nourish your soul by reading other supportive literature (see Appendix II for some ideas). You'll feel a shift from within. Suddenly, your soul will feel lighter and freer than ever before, even amidst adversity.

*How much does your soul weigh?*

My soul feels light and free. And yet, I sense I am only beginning to grasp what this really means. As the author of this book, I have lived this journey of freedom longer than any of my clients, workshop participants, or readers like you. As such, you might think I am an "expert," that I have "arrived," that I am a "master." However, I am always learning more. Writing this book has allowed me to experience the process of Intuitive Self-Care more deeply than I ever did before. By reviewing the entries in my journal,

I can look back to the way I was living a year ago and I see incredible changes. I am more accepting of myself and the events of my life. I am more in tune with my body's needs for food and exercise. I am more sensitive to my emotions and their messages. I am more aware of how to meet my needs and those of others. I am more faithful and trusting of my intuition. During my final edits, I found myself underlining passages that had real significance for me. I put these elements into practice more soulfully than ever, and now additional incredible changes are unfolding. I feel more happy, healthy, balanced, peaceful, and confident than I have ever been. I'm not just ACTING AS IF any more. I am *LIVING* AS IF. And you can—*will*—too!

*How much does your soul weigh?*

*LIVE AS IF* your soul is light and free. Experience the lightness and freedom of your soul, *all the time.* Instead of feeling a "split," in which you are either guided by the world or by your soul, imagine being a congruent extension of your core essence, *all the time.* How can you enjoy this? Let your soul guide your way. One of my obese clients, Shelley, is learning to LIVE AS IF by viewing her weight problem as her friend instead of her enemy. With this sense of acceptance *in each moment,* she converts any desire to overeat into a desire to nourish her body instead. I'm thinking back to the story I told you in the introduction to this book, about the phone call I received from the woman who called herself Shadow—and how her voice reflected the "dark places" in me, and in us all. LIVING AS IF involves transforming these "dark places" into "light places," which help you rather than hold you back. I liken this process to what happens when a light is turned on in a dark room—the darkness disappears, as if it has become the light. In his book *The Power of Now,* Ekhart Tolle shares a quote from

St. Paul that expands on this concept: "Everything is shown up by being exposed to the light, and whatever is exposed to the light itself becomes light." Are you ready for the next phase of your journey? Make the shift from *ACTING AS IF* to *LIVING AS IF.* Be who you really are. Let any obstacles become your opportunities. Experience your freedom on an ongoing basis. Let your soul shine radiantly. *Shadow, BE the Light* . . .

# self-test—

# how much does your soul weigh?

Getting a sense of the "weight" that is burdening your soul may seem difficult, so I developed this Self-Test to give you an estimate. I use this assessment during my workshops, and participants' feedback led to the development of the scoring system. You'll notice that your responses are multiplied by 10, or by 100 in some cases—the higher the multiplier, the more that particular question reflects a substantial load. For example, "losing those last ten pounds" can be the obsessive focus of your life. Therefore, in question 6, worrying about losing 1–10 pounds is multiplied by 100, while being concerned about losing 11–20 pounds is multiplied by 10, and trying to lose 21 or more pounds has no multiplier.

This assessment is not designed to provide you with the

actual "weight" of your soul—but it can offer you a perspective on the weight your soul has been carrying due to your various weight-loss efforts. So, give it a try.

## SELF-TEST: HOW MUCH DOES YOUR SOUL WEIGH?

*Directions: Provide a number in response to each question, multiplying your response as noted (i.e., × 10 means multiply by 10, × 100 means multiply by 100).*

1. On any given day, the number of times you worry about food, weight, exercise (× 10)    ___

2. The number of "games dieters play" (listed in Ch. 2) that you've tried (× 10)    ___

3. The number of other "diet rules" you have followed (× 10)    ___

4. How many years you've been trying to lose weight (× 10)    ___

5. The number of times you've lost weight, only to regain it (× 10)    ___

6. How much weight you'd currently like to lose (if 1–10 lbs., × 100; if 11–20 lbs., × 10)    ___

7. The total amount of weight you've lost and regained over the years    ___

8. The amount of money you've spent trying to lose weight    ___

9. How much money you'd be willing to pay for the "magic pill"  —

10. On a scale of 1 to 100, how important weight loss is to you (100 = extremely)  —

TOTAL SCORE:  —

*Scoring: Total all of the responses for each question, and write this number in the space provided for your total score. This gives an estimate of the "weight" that is burdening your soul due to your weight-loss efforts over the course of your entire life.*

0–99: Your soul is fairly light and free.

100–999: Your soul is moderately weighed down.

1,000 or more: Your soul is heavily burdened.

*Follow-up: To monitor your progress in losing the "weight" from your soul, take the self-test again in a month's time, modifying the questions appropriately (e.g., how many "games dieters play" that you've tried in the past month, how many days you've been trying to lose weight, etc.).*

# recommended reading

Throughout this text I have referred to several books that helped me on my journey of freedom. There are also many other resources that I have found helpful, and that I recommend to my clients. I've listed these resources in categories to facilitate your selection. Enjoy some additional reading to nourish your soul!

## FREEDOM FROM EATING DISORDERS AND THE DIET MENTALITY

Fodor, Viola *Desperately Seeking Self: An Inner Guidebook for People with Eating Problems* (Gurze Books, 1997)

Hall, Lindsey and Cohn, Leigh *Bulimia: A Guide to Recovery* (Gurze Books, 1986)

Hall, Lindsey and Ostroff, Monika *Anorexia Nervosa: A Guide to Recovery* (Gurze Books, 1999)

Harper, Linda R. *The Tao of Eating: Feeding Your Soul Through Everyday Experiences with Food* (Innisfree Press, Inc., 1998)

Hirschmann, Jane and Munter, Carol *Overcoming Overeating* (Fawcett Columbine, 1998)

Johnston, Anita *Eating in the Light of the Moon: How Women Can Transform Their Relationships with Food Through Myths, Metaphors and Storytelling* (Gurze Books, 1996)

Kano, Susan *Making Peace with Food: Freeing Yourself from the Diet/Weight Obsession* (Harper & Row Publishers, 1989)

Pipher, Mary *Hunger Pains: The Modern Woman's Tragic Quest for Thinness* (Ballantine Books, 1995)

———— *Reviving Ophelia: Saving the Selves of Adolescent Girls* (Ballantine Books, 1995)

Roth, Geneen *Breaking Free from Compulsive Eating* (Signet, 1984)

Sandbek, Terence *The Deadly Diet: Recovering from Anorexia and Bulimia* (New Harbinger Publications, Inc., 1986)

Siegel, Michele; Brisman, Judith, and Weinshel, Margot *Surviving an Eating Disorder: Strategies for Family and Friends,* revised and updated (HarperCollins Publishers, 1997)

Tribole, Evelyn and Resch, Elyse *Intuitive Eating: A Recovery Book for the Chronic Dieter* (St. Martin's Press, 1995)

## IMPROVING BODY IMAGE

Hirschmann, Jane and Munter, Carol *When Women Stop Hating Their Bodies: Freeing Yourself from Food and Weight Obsession* (Fawcett Columbine, 1995)

Hutchinson, Marcia Germaine *Transforming Body Image: Learning to Love the Body You Have* (The Crossing Press, 1985)

Johnson, Carol A. *Self-Esteem Comes in All Sizes: How to Be Happy and Healthy at Your Natural Weight* (Doubleday, 1995)

# OVERALL HEALING OF THE SOUL, MIND, AND BODY

Gawain, Shakti *The Four Levels of Healing: A Guide to Balancing the Spiritual, Mental, Emotional, and Physical Aspects of Life* (Nataraj Publishing, 1997)

Hay, Louise *You Can Heal Your Life* (Hay House, 1984)

Louden, Jennifer *The Woman's Comfort Book: A Self-Nurturing Guide for Restoring Balance in Your Life* (HarperCollins Publishers, 1992)

Markova, Dawna *No Enemies Within: A Creative Process for Discovering What's Right About What's Wrong* (Conari Press, 1994)

Myss, Caroline *Anatomy of the Spirit: The Seven Stages of Power and Healing* (Harmony Books, 1996)

—— *Why People Don't Heal and How They Can* (Harmony Books, 1997)

Northrup, Christiane *Women's Bodies, Women's Wisdom: Creating Physical and Emotional Health and Healing* (Bantam Books, 1994)

# PERSONAL GROWTH AND SPIRITUAL ENRICHMENT

Borysenko, Joan *A Woman's Journey to God* (Riverhead Books, 1999)

Chopra, Deepak *The Seven Spiritual Laws of Success: A Practical Guide to the Fulfillment of Your Dreams* (New World Library, 1994)

Dyer, Wayne W. *Manifest Your Destiny: The Nine Spiritual Principles for Getting Everything You Want* (HarperCollins Publishers, 1997)

—— *You'll See It When You Believe It: The Way to Your Personal Transformation* (Avon Books, 1989)

—— *Your Sacred Self: Making the Decision to Be Free* (HarperCollins Publishers, 1995)

Gattuso, Joan *A Course in Life: The Twelve Universal Principles for Achieving a Life Beyond Your Dreams* (Jeremy P. Tarcher/Putnam, 1998)

Gawain, Shakti *Creative Visualization* (New World Library, 1995)

—— *Developing Intuition: Practical Guidance for Daily Life* (New World Library, 2000)

Millman, Dan *The Laws of Spirit: Simple, Powerful Truths for Making Life Work* (H.J. Kramer, Inc., 1995)

Moore, Thomas *Care of the Soul: A Guide for Cultivating Depth and Sacredness in Everyday Life* (HarperCollins Publishers, 1992)

—— *The Re-Enchantment of Everyday Life* (HarperCollins Publishers, 1996)

Mundy, Jon *Listening to Your Inner Guide* (The Crossroad Publishing Company, 1995)

Redfield, James *The Cellestine Prophecy: An Adventure* (Warner Books, Inc., 1993)

Robinson, Lynn *Divine Intuition: Your Guide to Creating a Life You Love* (Dorling Kindersley Publishing, Inc., 2001)

Tolle, Ekhart *The Power of Now: A Guide to Spiritual Enlightenment* (New World Library, 1999)

Walsch, Neale Donald *Conversations with God: An Uncommon Dialogue, Book 1* (G.P. Putnam's Sons, 1996)

Williamson, Marianne *A Return to Love: Reflections on the Principles of a Course in Miracles* (HarperCollins Publishers, 1992)

Zukav, Gary *The Seat of the Soul* (Fireside Books, 1990)

Zukav, Gary and Francis, Linda *The Heart of the Soul: Emotional Awareness* (Simon & Schuster, 2001)